MEDICAL CANNABIS IN CANADA

FROM HISTORICAL LOWS TO THE CURRENT HIGH

MARK H. KIMMINS, MD

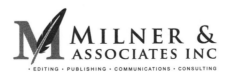

MILNER & ASSOCIATES INC
· EDITING · PUBLISHING · COMMUNICATIONS · CONSULTING ·

ISBN 978-1-988344-17-1 (paperback)
ISBN 978-1-988344-18-8 (e-book)

Production Credits
Editor: Andrea Maxie
Proofreader, publisher, and project manager: Karen Milner, Milner & Associates Inc.
Interior design and typesetting: Adrian So, AdrianSoDesign.com
Cover design: Adrian So, AdrianSoDesign.com

Printer: Friesens

Published by Milner & Associates Inc.
www.milnerassociates.ca

Printed in Canada
10 9 8 7 6 5 4 3 2 1

To all the Canadians who worked long and hard to remove the stigma around cannabis, and to my family who supported and tolerated the process of writing this book.

CONTENTS

INTRODUCTION

This book is about medical cannabis in Canada, and I hope it will serve as a useful guide for Canadian patients and health care providers. It's about the journey from complete prohibition and stigma to full legalization, and it will discuss how Canada emerged as a world leader in the field. It traces the history of medical cannabis over thousands of years to where we are today and predicts where we are heading in the future. It tells the story of a remarkable plant that not only produces numerous unique chemical compounds of medicinal value but is also increasingly being accepted as a recreational relaxant and euphoriant.

I discuss the cannabis plant itself and where its medicine comes from, and I explain how the plant medicine works within our bodies to produce its effects. I review the science underlying the plant's medical effects and evaluate the evidence supporting its use in a wide variety of disease. I also explain the difference between recreational cannabis and medical cannabis and provide guidance to Canadians looking for more information on the specific medical applications of the plant.

Within the text, you will find a discussion of the laws and regulations guiding current use and advice on how to navigate the current system as a patient. Finally, the book provides a lot of practical information on how to use cannabis medicine, including a discussion of an approach to delivery methods, dosing, and safety considerations.

Cannabis has suddenly become very popular, and in 2019 it appears that we are witnessing the discovery of a new medicine. The seemingly sudden emergence of medical cannabis in Canada, the United States, Australia, Israel, and countries throughout Europe gives a sense that we are finally discovering the therapeutic potential of this remarkable plant. The reality, though, is that human beings have been interacting with this natural medicine for thousands of years. The famous scientist and educator Carl Sagan once postulated that cannabis may have been the first domesticated agricultural crop. The plant itself evolved and developed over millions of years in central Asia, and we have evidence of human habitation in that same part of the world for more than fifty thousand years. Therefore, it's reasonable to speculate that human-cannabis interaction goes back much further than we are able to prove.

Anthropological evidence shows human use of cannabis for fibre, food, oil, medicine, recreation, and religion for at least ten thousand years. For most of human history, the separation of cannabis into distinct recreational and medical categories was not relevant. Just as west coast native people used the cedar tree in almost all aspects of their lives, ancient people in Asia used the cannabis plant. Even today, the lines between recreational and medical cannabis can be blurry, a situation that presents both challenge and opportunity. The prohibition of cannabis over the last hundred years was really a brief aberration, but it lasted long enough to affect the beliefs and attitudes of anyone alive today. After a century of stigma, our science, culture, and political policy are finally coming together to allow this remarkable plant to re-emerge.

Canada, and particularly western Canada, has been at the forefront of pro-cannabis culture since the 1960s. Back then, no specific medical products were available, so while many people were self-medicating, the emphasis was on recreational use. For years, British Columbia–grown cannabis would win prizes in international cannabis competitions. Having grown up on Canada's west coast, I was exposed to cannabis use as part of everyday life decades before the current "green rush" started. Cannabis, while still technically illegal, was effectively decriminalized in British Columbia when I was a teenager. Use was so common that Vancouver police were far more likely to ask you to put out a joint than to arrest you.

Interestingly, I remember as a teenager observing both recreational and medical use. I knew doctors, lawyers, judges, and police officers who used cannabis as others would use a glass of wine. I knew older professionals who baked cannabis into edibles that they used for aches and pains, and insomnia. This culture slowly and ultimately led to cannabis cafés and dispensaries being so common in the province that enforcement was really no longer an option. For years, visitors to Vancouver would understandably be confused about the proliferation of visible and accessible cannabis stores, long before intended federal legalization was discussed. Now that cannabis is legal both medically and recreationally, the ultimate fate of these many unregulated dispensaries is still unclear. The larger and more established dispensaries are scrambling to become compliant, licensed, registered businesses. Currently, some British Columbian communities fear that "big corporate cannabis" will push out the large number of existing local growers who have been operating in the province for decades. How this situation will ultimately play out is unknown as provincial and municipal cannabis regulations are still evolving.

Much of the relaxed Canadian attitude toward cannabis started in the 1960s when tens of thousands of young people left the United States to avoid mandatory military service during the Vietnam War. Labelled draft dodgers, this group of young, peace-loving, and often academic individuals settled across Canada, particularly in coastal British Columbia. The group has been described as one of the largest and best-educated groups of immigrants ever received by Canada. These immigrants brought with them a pro-cannabis culture, cannabis seeds and plants, and pro-cannabis academic arguments that were the beginnings of the current cannabis revolution. Their arguments were validated by two scientific commission reports in the early 1970s, which both supported cannabis legalization or decriminalization but also clashed with the growing anti-drug politics of the time.

My personal journey into the world of cannabis started with exposure to the normalized mixed recreational and medical use in British Columbia and a nagging feeling that there was tremendous hypocrisy across North America in the enforcement of drug laws and the resulting consequences for individuals and communities. It simply did not make sense to me that people could go to jail for using something that seemed no worse than alcohol. It also did not make sense to me that I lived in a local culture where professional people were able to use the plant without fear of consequences, but in another area of Canada, people could lose their livelihoods for making the same choice. These persistent feelings resulted in my decision to choose "Why Cannabis Should Be Legalized" as the topic for my formal grade eight English essay, almost four full decades before federal legalization of cannabis in Canada.

Throughout my remaining high school and college years, my ongoing exposure was primarily to recreational cannabis. However, even then, I remember friends telling me they preferred cannabis over alcohol because it made them feel less anxious and socially awkward, indicating a possible cannabis effect beyond recreational euphoria. Despite current and past prohibitions on youth alcohol and cannabis use, I can't remember a party from those days where beer and cannabis were not present in equal measure. It was just part of life. Some of the most intelligent and successful students I knew were regular cannabis users. Among them are individuals who went on to become bank presidents, vascular surgeons, CEOs, RCMP officers, business owners, and politicians. I also knew my share of cannabis stoners and dropouts. People who, in modern terms, likely had developed a cannabis use disorder. In my experience, responsible cannabis use was common and normal. Problems with misuse were uncommon but did occur.

My cannabis story may very well have stopped when I was still a young adult; my exposure to cannabis became less and less frequent as I progressed through the arduous process of becoming a physician and surgeon. During my fourteen years of post-secondary education, I had almost no formal training about cannabis except for one day of related lectures in a fourth-year pre-med neuropharmacology course. I had a total of zero hours of training on the medical uses of cannabis during either medical school, residency, or fellowship. Interestingly, around the same time I was in medical training, some of the most important and fundamental discoveries of the endocannabinoid system were being made.

Despite those discoveries, more than two decades would pass be-fore I truly understood the potential and importance of the interaction between the cannabis plant and our internal cannabinoid system. During eight years of academic medical work in Seattle, I had no for-mal exposure to medical cannabis use by patients or physicians and hadn't yet even heard of the endocannabinoid system. In fact, I had almost no exposure to even recreational use by colleagues, as federal law in the United States at that time meant any direct contact with cannabis was a violation of US Drug Enforcement Administration and Centers for Medicare and Medicaid Services regulations, compliance with which is required to work as a licensed physician. Those federal barriers continue to prevent widespread acceptance of cannabis medi-cine by mainstream physicians in the United States. While widespread adoption of medical cannabis has also been slow in Canada, citizens have had the legal right at a federal level to use cannabis medicine since 2001. Many US states attempted decriminalization as far back as the 1970s, but the US federal government hasn't yet budged. This fundamental difference in federal cannabis laws has allowed Canada to pull away from the United States and distinguish itself as a medical cannabis leader in both North America and the world.

In terms of exposure to cannabis as formal medicine, it wasn't until 2014 while working as a surgeon in Alaska that my professional experience began. Despite ongoing federal prohibition in the United States, between 2010 and 2015 a tidal wave of state ballot measures was sweeping up and down the west coast of the United States, re-sulting in various forms of state-related cannabis legalization. At that time, Canada had already established the rights of Canadians to ac-cess medical cannabis, though the current legal medical cannabis framework that exists today was still evolving.

In 2014, a ballot measure legalized recreational cannabis use in Alaska for the third time. Initial attempts in 1975 and 2003 had been reversed after brief periods of legalization. As cannabis became normalized in Alaska again, more and more of my patients felt com-fortable discussing their use with me. I began to notice that patients who used cannabis were asking for fewer refills of opioid medication and that some of my Crohn's disease patients were reporting fewer flares. Two particular cases really got my attention. One was a man who returned his unused Percocet prescription after a particularly painful surgery and used only cannabis while recovering. The other case was a young woman who avoided surgery after her Crohn's fistulas healed while using cannabis and no other medicines. While anecdotal, these cases seemed important and started my serious focus on the potential use of cannabis as a legitimate medicine.

The final deciding factor for me was direct observation of the profound palliative benefits of cannabis in my own father after diagnosis and treatment of glioblastoma brain tumour. This particularly aggressive form of brain cancer is also quite common, and it's the cancer that killed musician Gord Downie and senator John McCain. Suffering from the common and disabling side effects of chemotherapy-induced nausea and vomiting, my father could not eat and was becoming weaker and more debilitated. He was not responding to commonly prescribed anti-nauseants and was given cannabis by a friend. Not only did his nausea abate with cannabis, but his appetite also increased and he was able to get out of bed to eat. These changes resulted in a positive vicious cycle of improved ambulation and strength, improved sense of well-being, and recovery from the side effects of cancer treatment. I can't say with any scientific certainty that cannabis is a primary reason my father remains one of the longest survivors on the Canadian glioblastoma cancer registry, but I can say with certainty that it contributed to his remarkable recovery and to his quality of life during the worst days of his illness.

These experiences are how my official journey into the world of cannabis medicine began. Looking back, it almost seems like the path was predestined. While I would like to claim amazing prescience and foresight, I believe the truth is that, like many, I am aware that cannabis has been recognized as a remarkable medicine for much of human history, that it should never have been criminalized, and that its re-emergence was inevitable. I hope this book will provide some useful insights into both the past history and the current status of cannabis as medicine in Canada.

At the time of writing, Canada has just become the first major Western democracy to fully legalize cannabis. Already, we've experienced growing pains as product shortages developed within days of legalization when demand outstripped supply. Provinces and municipalities continue debate on some issues, and there is still some uncertainty as to what the ultimate legislative and distribution framework will be at the local level. What now appears certain, however, is that Canada will continue to have distinct and separate medical and recreational streams. Health Canada has declared that the current medical cannabis legislation will remain in force for at least five years and that plant cannabis compounds will remain as prescription-only products with limited exceptions for recreational use. This framework should guarantee that Canadian patients who demand access to medically specific cannabis products through the advice and consent of licensed health care providers should be able to do so. Note that throughout this book, I use *health care provider* or simply *provider* as inclusive terms to refer to any medical practitioner who is licensed to prescribe medical cannabis in Canada. In addition to physicians, nurse practitioners can also prescribe in an increasing number of provinces, currently including Ontario, Manitoba, and Nova Scotia.

My hope is that this book provides an interesting and informative discussion of medical cannabis in Canada for most readers and presents enough data to satisfy the basic needs of those looking to become either patients or providers in this re-emerging field of medicine. While I've tried to balance the needs of a potentially diverse readership, some sections may be too general and non-academic for medical experts, and others may be a little too technical for those unfamiliar with medical terminology. I've provided a glossary of key terms to help guide readers who are unfamiliar with cannabis science, and I encourage expert readers to go back to the cited source material and delve deeper into the subject matter themselves. The book concentrates on the Canadian experience with medical cannabis, from history to current legislation, but at times I also explore a broader scope. Because the re-emergence of cannabis is a global phenomenon, I discuss US history that has influenced Canadian culture and policy and review research from around the world that is guiding medical practice. For all readers, I hope that you enjoy our discussion of the remarkable cannabis plant and find some of the material relevant for your specific intentions.

PART I
A BRIEF HISTORY OF CANNABIS

Human beings have been using cannabis for thousands of years. Observing the current rapid expansion of the cannabis industry and the fact that humans have been interacting with cannabis for most of our history, it's becoming difficult to remember how and why cannabis ever became so stigmatized. Numerous published books already trace the path of cannabis from its ancient prehistoric roots to the present day in detail. And while it's not the intention of this book to fully repeat the history of cannabis, some background may help to understand how we got where we are today. This section therefore provides an abbreviated history of cannabis and our relationship with this remarkable plant, giving specific attention to medical context and Canadian experience. Later in the book, I discuss the plant and its medical applications in more detail.

CHAPTER 1
ORIGINS AND EARLY HISTORY

The cannabis plant evolved millions of years ago on the plains of central Asia. Cultivation of the plant may go back fifty thousand years to when people first settled in that area, although we do not have proof of human use going back that far. The earliest evidence of possible cannabis use comes from archaeological sites in the Czech Republic dated 26,980 BCE to 24,870 BCE, where impressions of plant fibre cordage consistent with woven hemp were found in clay fragments on the floors of ancient dwellings.[1] While these Stone Age Czech settlements show possible use of the cannabis plant in ancient eastern Europe, more solid anthropological evidence strongly suggests deliberate use since at least 10,000 BCE in Asia. In either case, evidence shows that humans have been using and cultivating cannabis for more than ten thousand years, making cannabis one of the first cultivated agricultural crops. In this chapter, I take a closer look at the origins and early uses of the cannabis plant.

FROM ORIGIN TO CULTURAL INTEGRATION
Despite the early Czech findings, most scientific evidence suggests that cannabis plants originally evolved on the steppes of central Asia, near what is now Mongolia and Siberia. Evidence for some of the earliest human settlements was found in this same geographical area. Therefore, since early humans and the original plants

co-existed in the same place, cannabis seeds and plants likely spread from central Asia along traditional trade routes and with nomadic tribes. Paleobotanical evidence of cannabis—such as pollen grains, fibres, seeds, plant impressions, trichomes (the glandular hair-like outgrowths found on cannabis flowers), carbonized remains, and cannabinoid compounds—has been recovered from dated archaeological sites throughout Asia and Europe along these trade routes,[2] suggesting steady spread from the area of origin. Much of this early archeological evidence is of fibre, rope, cloth, and jars of seeds, suggesting that prehistoric people primarily used cannabis plants for food, shelter, and clothing. The plant's versatility resulted in widespread cultivation of cannabis, again with emphasis on fibre, rope, and cloth production, throughout Europe, Asia, and even North America.

While evidence from the southern hemisphere is not as well documented in Western literature as the historical records from Asia and Europe, evidence suggests that cannabis did, ultimately, spread throughout most of the world. From Asia and the Middle East, the plant migrated into North Africa and from there appears to have become widely established throughout the African continent by the 1500s. In the western southern hemisphere, traders arriving in South America from Europe likely brought seeds and plants to South America on trade ships. Once again, hemp was the primary varietal of the cannabis plant that became widely established as an agricultural crop throughout much of the world. As a result of adapting to different growing conditions around the world, the cannabis plant developed a number of different varietals, also called *strains* or *cultivars*. (I discuss these further in Chapter 4.)

Ancient Chinese documents serve as some of the best records of early human cannabis use, detailing widespread use of the fibre-predominant hemp varietals for making rope, fabric, paper, fishing nets, and building materials. Evidence shows the ancient Chinese Yangshao culture (5000 BCE to 3000 BCE) extensively grew and used cannabis in everyday life.[3] The Yangshao people clothed themselves with hemp fabric, strung their bows with hemp fibre, wrote on hemp paper, and, ultimately, used hemp as medicine. An early Chinese surgeon even used an alcohol-based cannabis extract as an anaesthetic for surgeries.

While China was the source of some of the best and most extensive documentation of cannabis use, the plant was integrated into cultures throughout Asia, including India, Korea, and Japan. However, few nations integrated cannabis use into daily life as thoroughly as India. This integration was due, in part, to widespread acceptance of cannabis by religious leaders and scholars. The *Atharva Veda* (a collection of Indian religious texts) reportedly mentions cannabis as one of five sacred plants, referring to it as a "'source of happiness,' 'joy-giver,' and 'liberator.'"[4] Indeed, in some parts of the world, cannabis is still known as "the sacred plant." Reportedly, the Indian god Shiva took shelter under a cannabis plant and consumed it as food. Hence, cannabis use became widely incorporated into numerous religious rituals in the Indian subcontinent. For centuries, Indians have used bhang, a sort of cannabis milkshake, as a recreational relaxant and euphoriant. Recreational bhang use was traditionally as common as alcohol is in Western countries and was used as ubiquitously and in much the same way—to relax, relieve anxiety, provide social lubrication, and offer hospitality. Bhang use has been so integrated and widespread in India that the Lord Shiva is also known as the Lord of Bhang. It's still used widely in India today.

DISCOVERY OF MEDICINAL PROPERTIES

While much of the anthropological evidence suggests early primary use of cannabis plants for shelter and clothing, a significant written record also reveals specific medical cannabis use going back more than five thousand years over multiple cultures and civilizations. Discovery of the medicinal and psychoactive properties of the plant likely came through ingestion of a cannabis varietal that happened to produce more active chemicals. Female cannabis plants adapt to warmer climates by producing more abundant resin in glands, called trichomes, on their flowers. This resin contains the concentrated medicinal and psychoactive chemicals. One of the main traditional cannabis food sources was cannabis seeds, produced by female plants, which would normally contain only trace quantities of psychoactive chemicals. But because the seeds are located within the plant's flowers where the resin is produced, people probably would have occasionally ingested flowers and resin along with seeds. Therefore, it was likely ingestion of the flowering parts of adapted female cannabis plants that led to the discovery of the plant's psychoactive properties. Although, as I explain in Chapter 4, raw cannabis is not particularly bioavailable as a medicine or psychoactive agent, people probably discovered both properties by eating large quantities of flowers and seeds from these adapted plants. As different varietals of the cannabis plant contain variable quantities of chemicals, ancient people likely discovered medicinal uses for both the psychoactive and non-psychoactive forms of the plant over time.

Medical use of cannabis was well documented throughout Eastern regions of the world during the three millennia between 3000 BCE and early CE. Ancient Chinese scripts describe medical cannabis use in detail, and the oldest published Chinese pharmacopeia, the *Shennong Bencaojing*, mentions multiple medicinal uses of the plant, including use for menstrual cramps, rheumatic pain, and dementia.[5] The history of medicinal cannabis in China includes descriptions by the famous surgeon Hua Tuo, who documented the use of a powerful anaesthetic made from cannabis and alcohol. Further west, Egyptian hieroglyphic and papyrus records dating between 2000 BCE and 1700 BCE document specific use of cannabis as a medicine to relieve pain and depression, and the Greek historian Herodotus described the use of both medical and recreational cannabis in steam baths in the fifth century BCE.[6,7]

While documentation of medical cannabis use can be found from Eastern civilizations as diffuse as the Carthaginian, Persian, Greek, Egyptian, and Roman Empires, it was likely the Chinese who were responsible for most early discoveries of medicinal use and, thankfully, they maintained the most extensive records. In the twenty-eighth century BCE, the legendary emperor and founder of Chinese medicine Shennong, or Shen Nung, formalized an approach to medicine that relied heavily on the use of medicinal plants. Shennong reportedly wrote the first Chinese pharmacopeia, called the *Shennong Bencaojing*, also known as the *Shen-nung Pen-ts'ao Ching* or, in English, *The Classic of Herbal Medicine*. The *Bencaojing* outlined medical applications of almost four hundred plants, including cannabis. More than fifty editions of this book were published over four millenniums between approximately 2700 BCE and 1600 CE.

Vignettes from the various versions of the *Bencaojing* highlight how the discovered psychoactivity of cannabis was variously regarded over Chinese history. Some later editions of the book indicate that ingestion of too much cannabis would induce visions of demons and suggest that prolonged ingestion would allow communication with spirits. Around 600 BCE, when Taoism started to flourish in China, intoxication from cannabis, or any source, was viewed with contempt. However, a few hundred years later, around 100 CE, practitioners of the same religion were curious about this dimension of cannabis use and deliberately used the psychoactive experiences derived from cannabis ingestion in an attempt to achieve enlightenment and immortality.

EVOLVING CANNABIS MEDICINE

While we have extensive writings documenting the use of cannabis as medicine in ancient Asia and the Middle East, the use of cannabis as a medicine in the West does not seem to have been common or well documented until much later. This apparent lack of medicinal use and associated documentation may be the result of the fact that, in contrast to cannabis grown in hotter climates, the varietals of cannabis that grow best in the colder and more northern climates of Western countries typically have lower concentrations of medicinal chemicals. These non-medicinal varietals of cannabis were traditionally known as hemp.

One of the earliest references to possible medical use in the West occurs in the writings of English scholar Robert Burton, who mentions hemp seeds as a possible cure for depression in his book *The Anatomy of Melancholy* in 1621.[8] Noted English botanist and physician Nicholas Culpeper in 1652 published *The English Physician* (now known as *Culpeper's Complete Herbal*) in which he described the use of hemp for pain and inflammation.[9] However, not until the plant was described and classified by early explorers and botanists, such as Carl

Linnaeus and Jean-Baptiste Lamarck in the 1700s, do we have specific references to medical cannabis in Western texts.

During the 1800s, medical cannabis started to flourish in the West. In 1821, British botanist and pharmacologist Samuel Frederick Gray published *A Supplement to the Pharmacopoeia: Being a Treatise on Pharmacology in General,* in which he stated that cannabis could be used to make "an intoxicating drink."[10] This remark suggests that by the early 1800s the psychoactive and sedative properties of medical cannabis were known in England and Europe. In France, Dr. Jacques-Joseph Moreau published *Hashish and Mental Illness* in 1845 in which he theorized that the psychoactive properties of cannabis could be used to both treat and understand mental illness.[11]

Ultimately, the Irish physician and explorer Dr. William O'Shaughnessy is credited with helping cannabis become more widely established in Western medicine. He travelled to India to work as a surgeon, and there he was exposed to the therapeutic potential of the plant. After observing the effects on local people, he undertook experiments by giving cannabis and cannabis extracts to both people and animals. Having convinced himself of the safety of the plant, he continued to conduct therapeutic trials on sick Indian patients with a range of illnesses, from pediatric convulsions to rheumatism and cholera. So convinced was Dr. O'Shaughnessy of the efficacy of cannabis medicine that in 1843 he published the influential paper "On the Preparations of the Indian Hemp, or Gunjah (Cannabis Indica): Their Effects on the Animal System in Health, and Their Utility in the Treatment of Tetanus and Other Convulsive Disorders." In this publication, he describes a series of careful dosing experiments and the positive and negative effects of the treatment on convulsive disorders.[12] He concluded that small doses were medically effective and avoided sedative side effects. Indeed, the drug's usefulness as an anticonvulsant was so clear that he donated to a local pharmacy "a large supply of Gunjah" for any local surgeon or hospital that should require its use.

A follow-up publication by Dr. O'Shaughnessy, titled *The Bengal Pharmacopoeia, and General Conspectus of Medicinal Plants*, dedicated a large chapter to cannabis medicine, and this research influenced generations of physicians and pharmacists.[13] Among these health care experts was Sir John Russell Reynolds, personal physician to Queen Victoria. The queen was reportedly given cannabis preparations to relieve menstrual cramps and headaches. In his paper on cannabis medicine, titled "On the Therapeutical Uses and Toxic Effects of *Cannabis indica*," in the prestigious *Lancet* journal in 1890, Sir Reynolds, the queen's physician, stated that "in almost all painful maladies I have found Indian hemp by far the most useful of drugs."[14]

Between the 1850s and early 1900s, global attitudes toward cannabis began to shift toward the negative, but these perceptions made little difference to the plant's growing use and cultivation. Interest in cannabis medicine exploded, and cannabis products became common in doctors' offices and pharmacies. In 1893, the British Government established the Indian Hemp Drugs Commission whose findings ultimately spurred a thriving North American medicinal cannabis industry.[15] Though the commission was founded due to concerns about extensive use of bhang in Britain's Indian colony, it determined that cannabis use was attended by practically no harmful results. Subsequently, in the late 1800s and early 1900s, multiple large established pharmaceutical companies, including Bristol-Myers Squibb and Eli Lilly, were marketing, growing, manufacturing, and distributing medical cannabis products throughout North America. Pharmacies dispensed topical formulations, tinctures, gelcaps, and tablets aimed at treating a wide range of ailments and conditions. Had prohibition not occurred, cannabis medicine would almost certainly still be considered standard traditional medicine today.

CHAPTER 2
PROHIBITION ERA

Despite widespread medical use and little evidence of harmful side effects, countries around the world moved to prohibit cannabis use and cultivation in the early twentieth century. Even in India, where use of cannabis-containing bhang was widespread for centuries, moves were made to partially prohibit the plant. This prohibition occurred despite all available scientific evidence of the time pointing to the safety and usefulness of the plant. So when we examine the widespread international criminalization of cannabis, we therefore need to look beyond science to factors including the prohibitionist mindset, economic interests, racial prejudice, and anti-immigration sentiment to explain why prohibition occurred in various parts of the world.

The push back against cannabis had cultural and moral underpinnings and was at least partly a response to the perceived immorality of "loose" behaviour associated with recreational use. Much of the impetus for both alcohol and cannabis prohibition movements in Europe and North America came from the moral convictions of increasingly pious religious groups. And while alcohol prohibition ultimately failed, successful cannabis prohibition had many of the same origins and resulted in a push against cannabis in the US and Canada.

In the late 1700s and early 1800s, the temperance movement, a social movement against alcohol and inebriation, developed in many English-speaking countries, particularly in Canada and the US. The movement's origin was primarily various church denominations that began to speak on the immorality of drunken behaviour. Canada's first temperance societies emerged in the 1820s, and by the 1870s, hundreds of societies and church groups began to organize and push for full alcohol prohibition. The formal prohibition of alcohol in Canada came in various stages, from municipal bans in the late 1800s, to provincial bans in the early twentieth century, and full national prohibition from 1918 to 1920. The temperance act in Ontario ran from 1916 to 1927, and while aimed at alcohol, its influence spread to other inebriants. It was primarily these prohibitionist sentiments toward any and all inebriants that resulted in prohibition of cannabis in Canada in 1923. By the early 1920s, several US states had also started moving against the drug. However, by completing a countrywide prohibition in 1923, Canada became one of the first countries to make using cannabis illegal federally. The United Kingdom followed shortly after, prohibiting cannabis use in 1928. Federal legislation banning the plant in the United States, however, did not emerge until 1937. The global anti-cannabis effort culminated many years later in the United Nations Convention on Narcotic Drugs in 1961.

ONSET OF PROHIBITION IN CANADA AND THE UNITED STATES

In early twentieth century Canada, many people likely knew a physician who prescribed cannabis tinctures and remedies, but very few would have identified themselves as cannabis consumers, and recreational cannabis use was extremely uncommon. Therefore, the exact reason for cannabis criminalization in this country is somewhat mysterious and not very well known. Catherine Carstairs, a University of Guelph professor, wrote the book *Jailed for Possession: Illegal Drug Use, Regulation and Power in Canada, 1920–1961* and claims no one is sure exactly why cannabis was suddenly made illegal in Canada.[16] The timing, though, corresponds with the growth of the temperance movement, and it appears to have been mostly an issue of morality. The federal ban on cannabis in Canada came during the height of alcohol prohibition in Ontario, Canada's most populated province.

Formal narcotic prohibition in Canada began earlier than alcohol prohibition, with the Opium Act of 1908. In 1923, Prime Minister William Lyon Mackenzie King's Liberal government expanded it to the Act to Prohibit the Improper Use of Opium and Other Drugs. Previously, the only drugs on the schedule were opium, morphine, cocaine, and eucaine. A proposal to add heroin was widely agreed upon. Only a few weeks before the bill was introduced to Parliament, "Cannabis indica (Indian hemp) or hasheesh" was added to the list. The ban appears to have passed without discussion or debate, and why cannabis was added to the banned list does not seem to have been recorded. The bill passed and Canadian legislators successfully outlawed cannabis in 1923. This change was likely not huge news for the average Canadian citizen in 1923. Given the drug's relative anonymity, few Canadians would have held strong opinions on the matter. In fact, the prohibition of cannabis passed Parliament without any mention in the newspaper, and, as mentioned, without any recorded parliamentary debate.

The story of cannabis prohibition in the United States, however, is much more complex, being tied not only to prohibitionist culture but also to a growing anti-immigration sentiment. This piece of history is relevant to our Canadian story as US politics and culture around cannabis throughout the twentieth century heavily influenced Canada's experience and our own policy. As mentioned, recreational cannabis use was uncommon in the United States in the early 1900s, but both medical and recreational cannabis use was widespread in Mexico. When the 1910–1920 Mexican Civil War forced more than a million Mexican immigrants across the southern US border as they fled civil strife, these refugees brought with them their culture and customs— one of which was recreational cannabis. With it came its Spanish name, similar to the now-familiar English word *marijuana.** Though

---

*   In the early 1900s, established medicinal products in both Canada and the United States were known as cannabis or Indian cannabis, and the term *marijuana* was unknown. Because of the cultural and political attitudes that became affiliated with this particular name, understanding the etymology of the term *marijuana* is important for recounting the prohibitionist history. The term originates in Mexican Spanish, although its exact etymology remains a subject of debate. Most historians document that Spanish-speaking refugees referred to the product as *mariguana,* but the original origin of the word is unknown. The Oxford English Dictionary suggests the term may have come from the Nahuatl (Aztec) word *mallihuan.* Some suggest the word *marijuana* may also have originated from a Spanish translation of the Chinese words *ma ren hua,* meaning hemp seed flower. Regardless of its exact origins, the foreign-sounding word became established.

recreational use was slow to spread through the United States, a disdain for the plant quickly grew that aligned with the prohibitionist, and often racist and anti-immigrant, mentality of the time.

After Spanish-speaking immigrants introduced recreational products, cannabis was deliberately rebranded by US politicians and prohibitionists as *marijuana*, interchangeably spelled as *marihuana* or *mariguana*. This new term was then used to aggressively rebrand the nature and effects of cannabis as southern US states grew uncomfortable with the volume of Spanish-speaking migrants arriving in their cities. The word was officially adopted in the United States upon passage of the prohibitionist Marihuana Tax Act of 1937. The term *marijuana* is now falling into disfavour given its racist history and the fact that the scientific name of the plant genus is *Cannabis*.

While multiple forces converged against cannabis in North America, the final push in the United States was largely the result of one powerful and influential person: Harry Anslinger. Anslinger was the person primarily responsible for building the racial bias and anti-immigration sentiment against cannabis. He was also an early alcohol prohibitionist and had worked for the US Treasury Department's Bureau of Prohibition during the days when alcohol was illegal (US alcohol prohibition ran from 1920 to 1933). Later named the founding commissioner of the Bureau of Narcotics, Anslinger remained the head of this federal department until 1962. In the 1930s, having failed in his effort against alcohol, and perhaps to give purpose to his government agency, he began a notorious campaign against cannabis, freely claiming that "marijuana" caused criminal insanity and stating repeatedly that it incited aggressive, violent, and deviant sexual behaviour.[17] Anslinger also frequently included racially based themes and claims in his anti-cannabis rhetoric, directly connecting non-white persons to cannabis use and its claimed association with sexual deviance and moral depravity. For the group that had pushed alcohol prohibition, these moral arguments were likely an easy sell since they essentially came from the original temperance movement playbook.

A number of scientifically inaccurate and profoundly racist statements have been directly attributed to Harry Anslinger. Among the factually inaccurate statements he reportedly made are "Marijuana is the most violence-causing drug in the history of mankind," and "The deadly, dreadful poison that racks and tears not only the body, but the very heart and soul of every human being who once becomes a slave to it in any of its cruel and devastating forms." Anslinger's hateful, racist statements include "Reefer makes darkies think they're as good as white men," and "The primary reason to outlaw marijuana is its effect on the degenerate races." Though a lack of primary sources precludes complete validation of these quotations, they were so widely reported that it's highly likely that Harry Anslinger was the direct source. Despite his documented racist tendencies, Anslinger remained as head of the Bureau of Narcotics for longer than anyone before or since. He served for thirty-two years and influenced the failed drug policies in both the United States and Canada for almost a century. In many ways, he was the father of the war on drugs and the origin of decades of flawed policy that led to significant harm to minority communities and society at large.

Unlike policy makers before him, Anslinger ignored the evidence supporting cannabis, including the findings of the Indian Hemp Drugs Commission and the more recent Panama Canal report. The Panama Canal report was commissioned in 1925 by the US Army, which was concerned with increasing marijuana use by soldiers and workers at the Panama Canal. The army's report stated that "marijuana use has no appreciable deleterious influence on individuals using it."[18] It further concluded that the deleterious effects of marijuana had been exaggerated, and it recommended that no formal restrictions be placed on the use of the drug. In addition to this evidence, prior to passing the 1937 Marihuana Tax Act, congress received testimony from the American Medical Association (AMA) that cannabis was not the dangerous product Anslinger claimed it to be and that the AMA endorsed the medical applications of the plant.[19] All evidence was ignored, and biased, ignorant rhetoric won the day. Almost one hundred years of complete cannabis prohibition in the United States began. Despite prohibition, patients across North America and the world continued to find benefit and relief of symptoms by self-medicating with cannabis, and, ultimately, the voice and demand of cannabis supporters would bring the plant's story full circle, back to legalization. First, however, cannabis would have to survive the all-out war on drugs.

WAR ON DRUGS

Cannabis prohibition did not culminate until 1971 when President Nixon declared drugs to be "public enemy number one."[20] This vilification of drugs, including cannabis, was the start of the war on drugs. When cannabis prohibition was at its peak, the war on drugs thrived and all moderate debate disappeared. Opposing voices on cannabis were as likely to be as fundamentalist as their counterparts, either extolling the virtues and benefits of cannabis without question or, alternatively, being entirely anti-cannabis with no consideration of evidence and research data.

This polarized atmosphere made it easier for rigid cannabis laws to be enforced and for scientific evidence to be disregarded. Between 1939 and 1972, three rigorous North American scientific reports on cannabis reached the same conclusion: the harms of cannabis were overemphasized and the benefits downplayed. Scientific findings regarding cannabis were ignored by politicians in both Canada and the United States, and the drug war not only continued but in fact accelerated. The results of increasing drug arrests were that more prisons were needed, and in the United States, the industry of incarceration for profit soared. By 2013, the United States held the record for the highest rate of incarceration in the world, and much of this incarceration was for drug arrests. In the United States, 716 per 100,000 people were behind bars, in contrast to 118 per 100,000 in Canada.[21] With only 5 percent of the world's population, the United States had 25 percent of the world's prison population. With these astounding statistics in mind, let's review how the war on drugs in North America developed and the scientific reports that went unheeded.

For the first few decades after prohibition, little further attention was paid to cannabis use throughout North America. Even though non-medical cannabis had been uncommon in the first half of the twentieth century, prohibition managed to curtail both recreational and medicinal use. In Canada, any cannabis use was rare until the

1960s. In fact, after the 1923 ban, more than ten years passed before the first cannabis-related arrest. Even in 1962, there were only twenty cannabis prosecutions. However, with the counterculture revolution and mass movement of anti–Vietnam War Americans into Canada came a significant expansion of cannabis use. Politics of the drug war accelerated as well, and by 1972, there were 12,000 annual arrests. In the year 2000, there were 66,274 cannabis arrests in Canada.

Although cannabis prohibition stemmed from the temperance movement and anti-alcohol sentiment in both Canada and the United States, this mentality was further supported in the United States by strong anti-immigrant sentiments along the southern US border. Many of the first states to ban cannabis (California, Texas, New Mexico, and Louisiana) were on the border with Mexico, and the anti-cannabis drive was in large part a push back against the immigrants who were using the drug. Similar fears were harnessed in both Europe and Canada, where drug use was increasingly associated with dark-skinned races.

Starting with deliberate misinformation campaigns in the 1920s and 1930s, widespread dissemination of false and unscientific information instilled fear and skepticism regarding cannabis into the minds of North Americans. A well-known example is the 1936 propaganda film *Reefer Madness*, which tells a fictional tale of innocent white teenagers who descend into insanity, violence, and deviant behaviour after trying cannabis.[22] Deliberate propaganda like this film made calm intellectual debate about the pros and cons of cannabis virtually impossible for decades. Despite the predominant anti-cannabis culture, attempts at a scientific approach to the issue of cannabis safety were made. The three scientific groups that reviewed the benefits and harms of cannabis—the La Guardia Committee, the Le Dain Commission, and the Shafer Commission—each recommended decriminalization.

The La Guardia Committee was established in 1939 by the New York Academy of Medicine at the request of Mayor Fiorello La Guardia of New York City. The committee, composed of eight physicians, one psychologist, and four New York City health officials, studied cannabis smoking under both natural conditions in the city's tea pads

(rooms or apartments where people would gather to smoke cannabis in a social setting) and controlled conditions in the laboratory. It
also examined the potential link between cannabis and criminal behaviour. The study ran for five years and was published in 1944. The
conclusions of the committee were overwhelmingly pro-cannabis.[23]
The report remains a compelling historical document and the first
in-depth study of cannabis use in the United States. The La Guardia
committee's findings allegedly enraged Henry Anslinger as the report
rigorously and systematically contradicted claims he made regarding
the potential of cannabis use for causing insanity, promoting delin-
quency and criminal behaviour, and leading to the use of other drugs
(the so-called gateway drug theory).

In 1969, at the height of the Vietnam War and the counterculture hippie movement, Canada established the Commission of
Inquiry into the Non-Medical Use of Drugs, commonly known as
the Le Dain Commission (so named after its chair, Gerald Le Dain,
dean of Osgoode Hall Law School). The commission's purpose was
to examine the potential public health consequences of increasing
recreational cannabis use, much of which had come across the border with anti–Vietnam War immigration from the United States. Its
report, published in 1972, generated surprise when the commission
unexpectedly recommended decriminalizing all drugs. Regarding
cannabis, the commission's unanimous opinion was that it should
be completely decriminalized, with a minority opinion also suggesting full legalization and a government-controlled framework for legal
distribution.[24]

Around the same time as the Le Dain Commission was at work,
US president Richard Nixon hoped to find previously unproven harms
of cannabis. The recently established Controlled Substances Act divided drugs into five levels, or schedules, but the placement of cannabis
within these divisions was initially unclear. A controversial decision
was made to list cannabis as Schedule I, a category reserved for the
most dangerous drugs that had no potential benefit and maximum potential harm. The attorney general to President Nixon, John Mitchell,
reportedly convinced Nixon that they needed proof to keep cannabis
listed in the most dangerous category. This need for evidence of harm

gave birth to the Shafer Commission, appointed by President Nixon and chaired by Pennsylvania governor Raymond Shafer.

The Shafer Commission started work in 1971 and published its findings in 1972. The extensive report of more than one thousand pages was a complete rebuke and rebuttal of the previous thirty-five years of cannabis prohibition. The report was one of the first to claim that no case of cannabis overdose death could be found and the first to find no evidence that cannabis contributed to the use of other drugs.[25] The Shafer Commission stated that cannabis use carried minimal risk to public health and recommended not only that cannabis be removed from the scheduled drug list but also that its use and possession be decriminalized.

The findings of all three of these investigations were dismissed and ignored by the ruling governments of the time. Anslinger, of course, ignored and dismissed the La Guardia report in 1944. The Shafer Commission findings were not only completely ignored by the Nixon administration in 1972, but the government continued in its conviction and made public announcements that "America's public enemy number one is drug abuse."[20] A year later, Nixon created the Drug Enforcement Administration (DEA), instated harsh new penalties for drug offences, and increased statements about the dangers of cannabis. The recommendation of the Le Dain Commission to decriminalize all drugs in Canada in 1972 also clashed with the newly formed DEA in the United States and the accelerating war on drugs. After talks between Richard Nixon and Pierre Trudeau, the Le Dain Commission report was also shelved by the Canadian government. Despite no one in government listening,* the reports were not a total waste as the unanimous conclusion of these commissions ultimately spurred the future movements to re-legalize cannabis.

It was almost thirty years later when the next formal attempts were made in Canada to follow the recommendations of the Le Dain Commission. Prior to this initiative, cannabis had been listed as a

---

* Another notable example of this disregard came in 1988, when a prominent DEA judge, Francis Young, wrote an opinion supporting the Shafer Commission's findings. Judge Young stated that "marijuana is one of the safest therapeutically active substances known to man. By any measure of rational analysis marijuana can be safely used within a supervised routine of medical care." The judge recommended that the DEA transfer marijuana from Schedule I to Schedule II, advice which of course went unheeded.

prohibited substance under the Opium and Drug Act of 1923, the Narcotic Control Act of 1961, and the Controlled Drug and Substance Act of 1996. On May 27, 2003, the Liberal government of Jean Chrétien introduced a bill to decriminalize possession of small amounts of cannabis. Possession of 15 g or less would have been punishable with a fine, while those possessing between 15 and 30 g would be either ticketed or arrested and criminally charged at the officer's discretion. Personal cultivation of up to seven plants would have also become a minor offense. The bill almost passed into law but died when Parliament ended the session without resolution. Similar to the Le Dain report's initial consideration, this bill's failure was largely attributed to pressure from the US DEA. An almost identical bill was introduced in 2004 by the Liberal government of Paul Martin, but this bill did not become law because the minority government was defeated in a non-confidence vote. After the Conservative Party victory in 2006, no further attempts were made to change the legal status of cannabis until the Liberal Party of Canada proposed federal legalization in 2012. Formal debate on the proposed Cannabis Act under the Liberal government of Justin Trudeau started in 2016.

SOCIAL JUSTICE REPERCUSSIONS

Cannabis prohibition has had many serious intended and unintended consequences. It left a devastating legacy that continues to cause problems, not just in Canada but around the world. Many of the social justice issues related to cannabis prohibition are interconnected, creating a ripple effect with serious results. However well intentioned, the war on drugs often resulted in disproportionate negative effects on poor and minority populations throughout North America. The marijuana possession charge alone helped to industrialize the criminal justice system in both Canada and America, with cannabis possession accounting for approximately half of all police-reported drug offences in 2016 and 2017, as reported by Statistics Canada.[26]

The same trend is true in the United States, where the American Civil Liberties Union analyzed cannabis arrests between 2001 and 2010. It discovered that marijuana accounted for over half of all drug arrests in the United States.[27] The data also revealed a consistent trend toward significant racial bias. Although cannabis was consumed equally by all demographics—including people from predominantly white, suburban neighbourhoods—black people were 3.73 times more likely to be arrested for cannabis possession than white people. The incarceration rate for black men in the United States is more than six times higher than for white men.[28,29] These findings are borne out in Canada also. A 2017 study reported in the *Toronto Star* found that black people with no history of criminal convictions were arrested three times more often by Toronto police for possession of small amounts of cannabis than white people with similar backgrounds.[30] This racial bias is destructive. It ruins communities, and it ruins individual human lives.

In Canada and the United States, the repercussions of failed drug laws have been dismal. Even under Justin Trudeau's Liberal government in Canada, more than twenty-two thousand people were charged with cannabis possession, and over two thousand were convicted between October 2015 and April 2017. The criminal record accompanying these convictions can negatively change lives, stifle opportunities, restrict travel, and impart a stigma that may be impossible to reverse. The repercussions of having to confess a criminal record to every future employer, border guard, or landlord may be devastating. The fact that the criminal charge is simply for possession of a plant that has been a natural medicine for thousands of years, and one which is becoming increasingly decriminalized around the world, makes these consequences even more disturbing. As a positive sign, in some jurisdictions where cannabis is being legalized, there is a move to expunge previous cannabis convictions. In California, a bill has passed that is set to clear the records of more than 200,000 people. In Canada, now that cannabis is legal, Canadians previously convicted of possessing under 30 g of cannabis will soon be able to file a formal application for a pardon.

Despite this positive news in the Western world, perhaps the most chilling example of modern cannabis prohibition comes from Singapore where, in November 2016, a Nigerian man was executed for bringing cannabis into the country. His name was Chijioke Stephen Obioha, and at the time of his death he was thirty-eight years old. In

April 2007, police found 2.6 kg of cannabis at Obioha's home. He was condemned to death a year and a half later on charges of drug trafficking. He was never convicted of a violent offense—the entirety of his crime lay in possessing and distributing cannabis.

Throughout most of the world, and particularly the Western world, attitudes toward cannabis are suddenly and rapidly changing. Yet, for those still affected, the pace of progress can be frustratingly slow. Obioha was hanged less than three years ago, and lives continue to be ruined due to enforcement of failed prohibitionist laws. Despite overwhelming evidence against its position, the US government stubbornly continues to classify cannabis as a Schedule I drug. This irrational reality can't continue for much longer. With the passage of recent ballot measures in the 2018 US midterm elections, some form of cannabis legalization now exists in thirty-three states. More than 80 percent of US citizens now live in a state where cannabis is legal. This situation may trigger further legal action in the remaining states, like the 2017 lawsuit brought against the DEA and the Justice Department on the grounds that Schedule I listing of cannabis is "so irrational that it violates the U.S. Constitution."[31] Now that Canada has followed Uruguay and become the second nation to fully legalize cannabis, Mexico is planning to follow suit, and much of the world will likely soon do the same.

CHAPTER 3

LEGALIZATION ERA

Canada first gave Canadians legal access to medical cannabis in 2001. Since that time, a wave of cannabis legalization efforts has swept the globe, and twenty-six countries now have some form of cannabis legalization. Though full legalization is currently present in only Canada and Uruguay, it's thought to be imminent in at least ten more countries, including Mexico, Australia, and the United States. Today, the full legalization of cannabis in Canada could not be more significant or relevant to the general population. Almost 50 percent of Canadians admit to having used cannabis at least once, and Canada has some of the highest levels of cannabis use by youth in the world.[32] One of the primary reasons that Canada moved to legalized cannabis was to try and reduce use by young people, and another was to keep cannabis out of the black market.

To measure the relevance of cannabis economically, consider that a recent Deloitte study estimated that the potential economic impact of legal cannabis in Canada could be as high as $22.6 billion a year when factoring in ancillary businesses, such as security, transportation, and tourism.[33] This number may even be low, as a recent estimate suggested Canadians spent almost $6 billion on cannabis in 2017,[34] which was well in advance of legalization or any established industry to support legalization. Once distribution channels are in place and a wider range of cannabis products are available, spending is estimated to skyrocket. The modern world has rediscovered the cannabis plant in a major way and has begun to embrace it both medicinally and recreationally. Much of this rapid shift toward embracing cannabis likely has to do with its being embraced by big business. The reality is that public opinion often follows the money.

PRECEDENT FOR MEDICAL LEGALIZATION IN CANADA

During the prohibition years, some Canadian physicians and patients understood the value of cannabis for treating a range of symptoms and ailments, like epilepsy, anxiety, and insomnia, but were forced to pursue this remedy against the law. Access to cannabis was restricted to the illegal street market, where it was difficult or impossible to ascertain the quality or even the type of cannabis being purchased. For simply using this medicine, patients ran the risk of fines and even imprisonment. Although there were rumblings for decades regarding the fundamental injustice of denying cannabis to those who claimed a medical need for it, this area of Canadian law did not come back under intense scrutiny until the late 1990s with the story of Terrance Parker.

Parker suffered from epilepsy, caused by a hit to the head by a swing at the age of four. Conventional therapies for Parker's epilepsy were unsuccessful, with one treatment after another proving ineffective. While still a child, Parker was given a range of potent conventional pharmaceuticals, such as Dilantin, Mysoline, and Librium. When he was only fourteen, he was brought into a children's hospital for surgery. He had a grand mal seizure in the recovery room, and afterward the seizures grew worse.

After multiple hospitalizations, often due to accidents caused by seizures, Parker began consuming cannabis. Initial exposure came from trying cannabis given to him by another patient at a mental health care facility, and at first, he tried using it only to relax. When he noticed almost immediate improvement in the rate and intensity of his regular seizures, his family physician encouraged him to keep a journal cataloguing its effects.

Seven years later, in 1987, he was arrested for possession of cannabis. By now, Parker was medicating with cannabis every day and achieving positive results. After his arrest, he was taken before a provincial court in Ontario, and, with the help of a savvy lawyer, was acquitted based on his obvious and provable medical need for cannabis. He became the first semi-legal cannabis consumer in Canada, and his victory represented a landmark ruling, which would eventually play a key role in revolutionizing Canadian cannabis law.

Unfortunately, Parker's legal troubles were not over. On July 18, 1996, Toronto police raided his apartment, discovering seventy-one cannabis plants. He was charged with possession, cultivation, and trafficking. His next trial would become an even more significant point of reference in Canadian cannabis law as his attorney based his defence on the Canadian Charter of Rights and Freedoms rather than on the specific issue of Parker's medical need.

In the historic *R. v. Parker* case in 2000, attorney Aaron Harnett specifically referenced section 7 of the Canadian Charter, which states that "everyone has the right to life, liberty and the security of the person and the right not be to deprived thereof except in accordance with the principles of fundamental justice."[35] The argument stated that by forcing Parker to choose between imprisonment and his health, he was being deprived of his constitutional right to life.[36] Broadening Parker's defence to include his fundamental rights as a Canadian had an enormous impact on Canada's cannabis laws.

When the judge overseeing the case ruled in Parker's favour, he effectively read down sections of the 1996 Controlled Drugs and Substances Act, specifically those areas that prohibited persons who possess or cultivate cannabis for their "personal medically approved use." When a subsequent appeal upheld the ruling of the lower court, the federal government was put on notice. The Controlled Drugs and Substances Act would need to be changed, and some allowance would need to be made for patients with a demonstrable need for cannabis, or the current laws would be unconstitutional and, therefore, invalid in courts throughout Canada. This 2000 ruling led directly to new legislation that would enshrine into law the constitutional right of Canadians to access medical cannabis. By so doing, Canada became the first major Western country to legalize medical cannabis.

EARLY MEDICAL CANNABIS REGULATIONS

In 2001, the Marihuana Medical Access Regulations (MMAR) were written into Canadian law. This law was Ottawa's first attempt to arrive at a solution to the problems inherent in Terrance Parker's case. While the R. v. Parker ruling established that individuals like Parker were in an impossible legal situation, no mechanism had yet been developed for them to access cannabis legally nor had direct, clear guiding provisions.

The MMAR allowed those suffering from severe conditions, like epilepsy, AIDS, multiple sclerosis, and cancer, to use cannabis by applying to Health Canada for a permit to grow plants in their own homes. Patients would be allowed to cultivate under a series of strict (some would say prohibitively strict) guidelines. A select few were allowed to purchase cannabis directly from companies licensed by Health Canada. These were the earliest days of companies we now know as licensed producers (LPs), companies licensed and regulated by Health Canada to grow and produce clean, pesticide-free medical cannabis products. For a few years, only one small LP existed: Prairie Plant Systems, a Saskatoon-based company that grew its product in an underground mine in Manitoba. In 2013 they formed a subsidiary, which ultimately led to the development of Canada's first major modern cannabis producer, CanniMed.

In the spring of 2003, the Supreme Court of Canada re-examined the components of the MMAR and found them unconstitutional as they were failing to provide a safe, reliable, legal supply of cannabis to those who needed it. In some ways, the early legislation actually fueled the illegal cannabis market because it was initially easier to purchase product on the black market than comply with the difficult and restrictive government guidelines. The federal government responded by tweaking the rules, making it slightly easier for would-be cannabis patients to gain access to seeds and expediting their processing times for Health Canada approval. Despite these stopgap measures, the original 2001 MMAR system ultimately failed to provide a robust and functional means by which Canadians could exercise their new legal right to access medical cannabis. It took another decade of rewrites and revisions before the next version of Canadian cannabis law came into place with introduction of the Marihuana for Medical Purposes Regulations (MMPR).

The MMPR was enacted July 2013 and came with several significant changes. By this time, Health Canada was having difficulty tracking the many legal home-growing operations throughout the country—not to mention managing the growing paperwork from increasingly numerous applications. Ottawa's solution, enacted with the MMPR, was to disallow growing at home and have all cannabis patients access their medicine through LPs. Thankfully, since introduction of the legal cannabis program in 2001, the LP program had slowly progressed, allowing patients to choose from a variety of legal, quality-controlled cannabis products. Further, physicians were now empowered, and potentially encumbered, to prescribe cannabis under conditions set by Health Canada and the College of Physicians and Surgeons in their own provinces. Under the MMPR law, the only legal way to access cannabis was to purchase dried cannabis directly from official LPs after obtaining an official authorization from a licensed medical doctor.

The new model attempted to accommodate the increasing demand for medical cannabis in Canada, but a few structural deficiencies remained. By completely eliminating the grow-at-home program, the MMPR essentially forced patients to purchase expensive medicine from government-regulated businesses. It also made it difficult for some cannabis patients to access sufficient quantities of medicine and manage their own medical needs. Further, patients were allowed to register with only one LP and were thereafter confined to that LP for the duration of their time as cannabis patients. Finally, the MMPR allowed purchase of only dried cannabis flower, which limited a patient's options to choose intake methods other than smoking—a problem for patients with lung conditions, anyone wishing to avoid the potential respiratory problems associated with smoking, or anyone wishing to take advantage of the potential benefits of oral cannabis ingestion. Therefore, despite being an improvement on the 2001 MMAR, these two components of the 2013 MMPR regulations (the cancelled grow-at-home program and the limitation to dried cannabis) were quickly legally challenged and successfully argued in the courts.

Other issues arose from the new MMPR regulations. The new law required patients to obtain authorization for medical cannabis, in the form of a signed medical document from their physicians. However, no mechanism or funding to provide physicians additional education on cannabis was provided. Physicians' groups, like the Canadian Medical Association (CMA), almost immediately pushed back. Health care providers, without the benefit of any formal cannabis education, were legally mandated to be the gatekeepers of this new industry. Suddenly becoming legally empowered to issue medical cannabis documents to patients, health care providers often faced immense challenges in taking on cannabis patients as time constraints and lack of cannabis education made doing so very difficult.

The huge pent-up patient demand for access to medical cannabis, combined with a shortage of providers able or willing to write authorizing documents, gave birth to dedicated, stand-alone cannabis clinics across Canada. While many of these clinics operated legally and ethically within the framework of the original MMRP, a large number of opportunistic and illegal operations also arose. Examples of illegal behaviour included charging patients for medical services that would normally be covered under provincial health plans, billing health plans without providing full medical assessment, and selling illegal cannabis products directly to patients. Legitimate medical cannabis clinics must operate under the legal, ethical, and regulatory framework of conventional health care. The presence of dedicated medical cannabis clinics continues to be a matter of debate, but as long as patient demand exceeds the supply of providers willing to authorize medical documents, they will continue to exist. This situation won't correct until more health care providers feel educated on, and comfortable with, medical cannabis.

CURRENT REGULATIONS

Ultimately, the attempts of the both the MMAR and MMPR to regulate the emerging medical cannabis industry in Canada became the foundations of Canada's Access to Cannabis for Medical Purposes Regulations (ACMPR), introduced in 2016. The ACMPR regulations not only established parameters for legal, safe use of regulated medical cannabis in Canada and thereby delineated patient rights and responsibilities, but they also provided the legislative infrastructure for the recent legalization of recreational cannabis in the 2018 Canadian Cannabis Act. The ACMPR was the full legal framework for the production, distribution, sale, and possession of medical cannabis in Canada until October 17, 2018. While officially now replaced by the new Cannabis Act, Health Canada has declared that the basic rules and structure of the 2016 ACMPR will remain in place for medical cannabis until at least 2023.

The ACMPR rules differ from the 2013 MMPR legislation primarily in that they allow a grow-at-home program and also allow Canadians the right to purchase cannabis extracts in the form of oils in addition to dried cannabis flower. These changes occurred due to a number of successful court challenges arguing that forcing patients to purchase only dried flower from an LP caused undue financial hardship and unfairly forced patients to smoke cannabis or make their own edible extracts. Allowing patients to purchase edible oils significantly increased options for taking their medicine. The reinstatement of a grow-at-home program was also a critical change—the three-year reign of the MMPR may have been a short interval, but it was a long wait for patients who sought complete control over their medicine, who couldn't afford medical cannabis, or whose cannabis needs could not be met by the LP system.

In bringing back a grow-at-home program, Health Canada streamlined the application process and created additional options for patients. As well as allowing patients to grow their own cannabis themselves, the ACMPR allows patients to specify a designated grower, and multiple growing operations can be managed from the same site, provided everyone concerned has submitted a viable application and possesses a medical document issued by a licensed health care provider. Ultimately, this regulatory flexibility allows the needs of more medical cannabis patients to be met, including those of patients who require medical cannabis but can't afford it, or whose disabilities prevent them from growing their own.

The ACMPR also allows patient registration with more than one LP. This provision is meaningful to patients as, previously, producers would frequently have a shortage of supply, leaving patients without an alternative option. Furthermore, patients desired a wider selection of strains and cannabinoid products, and the ACMPR gives patients the option to choose a cannabis oil from one LP and a different dry cannabis product from another.

Under the ACMPR, LPs also have legislative relief that helps streamline patient registration. Previously, LPs needed to verify each medical document sent to them, creating potential communication chaos between the prescribing providers and the producers. Now, LPs can confirm a health care provider's signature, licence, and practice information once, and routinely accept medical documents from that person afterward, much the same way a pharmacy accepts prescriptions from known licensed providers. Health Canada also made it easier for LPs to operate by allowing a single application for production and sale of both fresh and dried cannabis, as well as cannabis oil and seeds. With the MMPR, an LP required an individual licence for each of these activities, making it challenging for LPs looking to diversify their products.

Under rules of the ACMPR, which are still in place, product testing is more stringent, routine, and reliable. LPs are now permitted to send cannabis to off-site accredited testing labs, which allows additional verification that the safety and quality of their products meet Health Canada's requirements. These requirements are essential to the functioning of a legitimate medical cannabis industry as products obtained from unregulated sources have unknown composition. Research also shows much of this illegal cannabis is contaminated. For example, a 2017 study found that more than 90 percent of product obtained from Southern California dispensaries was contaminated.[37] In addition to pesticides, other potentially dangerous contaminants in street cannabis include pathogenic moulds, viruses, synthetic additives, opioids, phencyclidine, and methamphetamine. Another recent study in California showed that over 80 percent of the cannabis concentrates and extracts available for sale at unregulated dispensaries contained potentially dangerous residual solvents, including isopentane, butane, heptane, and propane.[38] In Canada, and also now in California, all legal cannabis must be obtained from strictly regulated sources that follow the same good manufacturing practice regulations that apply to food, agricultural, and pharmaceutical industries. This requirement guarantees that products have been subjected to rigorous testing and standards and ensures that patients are accessing safe, medical-grade product instead of a potential slurry of unknown chemicals, pesticides, moulds, and other contaminants. While the Cannabis Act has now officially replaced the ACMPR, all safety and testing requirements of the ACMPR remain in place. I review the minor changes to the ACMPR under the Cannabis Act in the next section.

RECREATIONAL LEGALIZATION

Global perceptions of cannabis have once again shifted—this time to the positive—and a trend toward global cannabis legalization is rapidly developing. At the time of this writing, thirty-three countries currently have some form of cannabis legalization, two of which have full recreational legalization, and multiple other countries are set to follow soon. Legalization efforts are sweeping across Europe, Australia, and the Americas. Further east, reforms are slower, but already Thailand and South Korea have legalized medical cannabis. In India, where cannabis has a long history of acceptance in a religious context but was outlawed in the early 1900s, parliamentary debate on moving from traditional acceptance of bhang to full cannabis legalization began in early 2018. On October 17, 2018, recreational cannabis was officially legalized in Canada, making us the first major Western democracy to do so. The new Canadian legislation allows any adult to purchase and publicly possess up to 30 g of recreational cannabis at a time or grow up to four plants at a time for recreational use.

Many Canadians are wondering how recreational legalization will affect the medical cannabis patient. Cannabis is a unique plant, and there are currently no other examples of a naturally occurring medicine that also has safe recreationally intoxicating properties. The fact that it can be used both medically and recreationally has led some people, and some medical professional groups, to question whether separate recreational and medical streams should exist in Canada. The essence of their argument is that if cannabis is widely legally available for recreational use, why should patients have to see a health care provider, and why should providers have to give authorization for access?

The answers to these questions lie in the fact that medical cannabis products are not only specific and different from their recreational counterparts, but their intended uses and expected outcomes are also quite different. The intention of recreational customers is to achieve some degree of relaxation, euphoria, or high, and the expectation is that these effects are both desirable and anticipated. On the other hand, the intention of medical patients is to use a specific medical product to relieve symptoms or treat disease, and the expectation is that they will achieve relief without impairment or alteration of normal function. Only with the help of a health professional can appropriate risk-benefit medical treatment decisions be made. If health care providers are not involved, the only alternative would be to have medical patients self-medicate with products designed to produce an intoxicating recreational effect. This outcome would be considered unacceptable with any area of conventional medicine and is similarly unacceptable with cannabis medicine. Thankfully for the Canadian medical cannabis patient, Health Canada agrees.

In addition to maintaining the ACMPR framework and regulations for at least five years, Health Canada has stated that phytocannabinoids will remain as prescription-only products, with limited exceptions for recreational use. This provision means that plant chemicals extracted from cannabis will require a health care provider's authorization for use, with the exception of limited products available to the recreational consumer. Health Canada has also stated that employees in recreational cannabis stores will be prohibited from providing medical advice. These rules guarantee that the medical cannabis stream will continue uninterrupted after recreational legalization.

Health Canada has also made a few changes to the ACMPR that make accessing and using medical cannabis easier for patients. The ACMPR limitation that allowed purchase of only a 30-day supply of cannabis has been removed, and so have personal storage limits for cannabis in the home. Any adult Canadian is now allowed to store an unlimited amount of cannabis at home for either personal or medical purposes. Public possession limits for medical cannabis patients remain the lessor of one month's supply or 150 g of medical cannabis, in addition to the 30 g limit for recreational cannabis. Therefore, at the time of this writing, an official Canadian medical cannabis patient could carry 150 g dried cannabis or equivalent for medical purposes, plus 30 g dried cannabis or equivalent for recreational purposes.

Undoubtedly, the medical patient base will see some change now that all adult Canadians have legal access to recreational product. It's assumed that at least some medical patients may have been using the ACMPR to legally access cannabis for recreational use and that there will be some patient drop-off with recreational legalization. However, this inevitable small decrease in medical patient numbers will likely be offset by an increase in patients who were waiting until the product was fully legal before asking their health care providers for it. This shift is particularly true for the senior population and more conservative Canadians. Even though medical cannabis has been legal and available in Canada for years, these populations were still hesitant to access a product that was considered bad and illegal on the recreational side. Now that cannabis is fully legal, many of these patients feel it's ok to use. However, most of them have no interest, desire, or intention to access recreational cannabis. They want to see a physician for their medicine and receive a product intended for medical use. Requiring the senior population, or the pediatric population, to self-medicate with recreational product would be both immoral and likely medically ineffective.

Unlike recreational consumers, legitimate medical patients will have access to licensed health care professionals, will be eligible for compassionate medical pricing from LPs, and will often be able to obtain reimbursement of medical cannabis expenses. Additionally, the medical patient will likely be allowed tax deductions and use of medical benefits from employers or insurance when purchasing medical product. Also, depending on workplace policy, a health care provider's authorization may be necessary in order to consume cannabis medicine while employed. Finally, if unexpected shortages of cannabis plant material occur, priority access to available product will likely be given to those with a demonstrable medical need. None of these benefits will be available to recreational users.

For the medical market, there is increasing demand for new medicines from the many cannabinoid compounds that are not psychoactive. These products are not desirable or valuable as recreational products. Research, development, and marketing of these new medical cannabis products will depend on a separate legitimate medical cannabis market. Because Health Canada intends to keep the majority of cannabinoid products listed as prescription only, these new medicines won't be sold through recreational outlets. They will be strictly medicinal.

Overall, the effects of recreational legalization should be positive for the medical cannabis consumer. There will be less stigma and judgement toward users of cannabis, there will be more impetus for research to improve individual and community safety, and there will be an explosion of investment and research into way the cannabis plant and its products can be used to improve health.

PART II
CANNABIS AS MEDICINE

As discussed in Part I, the origins of medical cannabis likely go back before recorded human history began, and we have good evidence of human use for at least ten thousand years. Our current differentiation of cannabis into distinct recreational and medical categories would not have made sense to the early indigenous people. To them, the cannabis plant was a source of food, shelter, cloth, rope, and medicine, and it was also a recreational and religious euphoriant. We know that cannabis has been used as medicine for at least five thousand years, but description of the plant as specific medicine was not well documented until the early Chinese pharmaceutical texts. The trend to describe cannabis as medicine continued with the enthusiasm of European scientists to classify and categorize their natural world. Until recently, medical cannabis and recreational cannabis had significant overlap, and the separation was often based on the intent of the user. This lack of differentiation was mostly due to the fact that both recreational and medical users were using the same parts of the same plant.

In the 1800s and early 1900s, the booming pharmaceutical industry started to produce cannabis extracts and tinctures, which could be sold in forms that closely resembled other conventional medicines, like cough syrup, gelcaps, and tablets. Unfortunately, due to prohibition, these products went away for almost one hundred years. We are now entering a time when new medical formulations and delivery mechanisms are more sharply separating cannabis into distinct medical and recreational categories. For instance, a transdermal patch designed to give slow, steady delivery of a non-psychoactive cannabinoid for relief of arthritic pain is clearly very different from a pre-rolled cannabis cigarette sold to produce a recreational, psychoactive high. Legislation is also evolving that dictates how medical and recreational cannabis products must be produced, marketed, and sold using different rules and regulations.

It's only recently that we have begun to discover the underlying mechanisms by which cannabis works in our bodies. And it's only recently that we have had the technology to allow analysis and discovery of hundreds of potentially useful chemicals within the cannabis pant. This research brings with it the promise of a new age of cannabis medicine and also, potentially, plant medicine in general.

CHAPTER 4
THE CANNABIS PLANT

A basic understanding of the cannabis plant and its medical products is important for understanding medical cannabis use and applications. While a comprehensive and complete discussion of all aspects of the cannabis plant is beyond the scope of this text, more in-depth information is widely available in other publications for interested readers. What this chapter will cover are the necessary foundations for the prospective medical cannabis patient and provider.

CLASSIFICATION

Plants, like animals, are classified into categories, including family, genus, and species. The genus *Cannabis* is classified as a flowering plant in the family Cannabaceae, which includes trees (like the hackberry), vine-like plants (like hops), and herbs (like cannabis). Evidence suggests that cannabis evolved and separated from hops-like plants millions of years ago. The *Cannabis* genus is indigenous to central Asia and the Indian subcontinent, where researchers believe it has existed alongside human populations for more than fifty thousand years. The species part of the taxonomy, or classification, of cannabis plants is controversial. Some researchers believe that there are three distinct cannabis species while others believe there is only one true species with three to five sub-varietals. Most, however, agree that cannabis has two main varietals: sativa and indica.

In the original 1753 classification of the plant by noted botanist Carl Linnaeus, just one species was identified, *Cannabis sativa,* which is now known as *Cannabis sativa* Linnaeus. In 1785, biologist Jean-Baptiste Lamarck was given cannabis plant specimens collected in India. On the basis of several characteristics he observed that seemed different, including the shape of the leaves and flowers, Lamarck felt that these Indian plants should be distinguished from *C. sativa.* For these reasons, he named a new species called *Cannabis indica.* However, the differences in the Indian plants Lamarck observed may have been adaptations to a different environment rather than reflections of a different species. Debate on this matter continues to this day but, ultimately, is likely not relevant for the medical cannabis patient. Many researchers also acknowledge an uncommon third species, known as *Cannabis ruderalis*, that has low levels of medical and psychoactive cannabinoids. Note that just as we use the genus name, *Cannabis*, as the common name for the cannabis plant, we continue to use the species names of *C. sativa* and *C. indica* as common names for the traditional sativa and indica varietals. As I discuss later, these traditional names do not necessarily reflect the reality of modern medical cannabis plants, which are now mostly hybrids of original plant lineages.

CULTIVATION

Cannabis is a plant, and like any plant, it has nutritional and environmental requirements to grow. It can be grown indoors or outdoors. While one of its nicknames is *weed*, the plant required for production of medical products does not in fact grow as easily as most common weeds. Cannabis requires careful cultivation to maximize production of the plant's medicinal chemicals. Due to strict regulations stipulating quality control and lack of contamination, most Canadian LPs grow cannabis indoors in large greenhouses that take advantage of natural light and provide supplementary light as needed. Indoor growing allows for easier control of pests and pathogens and stricter control of environmental parameters.

ANATOMY: WHERE DOES THE MEDICINE COME FROM?

Many plants contain both female and male parts in their flowers, allowing them to self-pollinate. Cannabis, however, is dioecious, which means that it has separate male plants and separate female plants. Plants of both sexes are required for cannabis to reproduce, but only the female cannabis plant concentrates chemicals with medicinal properties in significant amount. Therefore, almost all cannabis medicine comes from the flowers of the female plant. In these flowers, concentrated chemicals are produced in glands called trichomes and stored in their resin, which is the source of cannabis medicine. These concentrated chemicals are used by the female cannabis plant to protect the reproductive organs from attack, to attract beneficial pollinator insects, and as part of normal plant metabolism.

Male plants, however, pose a problem for humans wanting to use these concentrated chemicals. Once pollen from the male plants reaches the flowers of the female plants, the female plants divert energy and metabolic pathways from flower growth, and hence trichome activity and chemical production, to make seeds. But if no pollination occurs, female plants continue to produce the resin and concentrate medicinal chemicals. To maintain this chemical production in female plants, male cannabis plants are manually eliminated from crops prior to developing pollen in traditional cannabis cultivation. In modern cannabis cultivation, seedless female plants are usually grown from clones of mother plants or from female stock generated from tissue culture in the lab. Male plants are typically only used as needed to generate new mother plants.

MEDICINAL COMPONENTS

The cannabis plant contains hundreds of chemical compounds, many of which have potential medicinal value. Research on some of these compounds is still in the early stages but is progressing rapidly in the new pro-cannabis environment. The primary categories of medicinally important chemicals are phytocannabinoids, terpenoids, and flavonoids.

Phytocannabinoids: THC, CBD, and Beyond

While the word *cannabinoid* refers to any molecule that interacts with our internal cannabinoid receptors, the word *phytocannabinoid* refers to any similarly functioning molecule produced specifically by the cannabis plant. (For the most part, though, I'll use the term *cannabinoid* inclusively unless having a focused discussion on phytocannabinoids, like in this paragraph, as *cannabinoid* is the most commonly used term.) Phytocannabinoids are hydrocarbon molecules that are metabolically active within the cannabis plant as part of normal plant physiology. These molecules, which we commonly refer to as chemicals or compounds, also work on our internal cannabinoid receptors, producing potential medicinal and therapeutic effects. As far as we know, the phytocannabinoids are unique to cannabis plants, and no other plants produce these exact chemical compounds.

While an individual cannabis plant may produce a hundred or more unique cannabinoid compounds, only a few of these are produced in any significant amount. By far the most well-known plant cannabinoid compounds are delta9-tetrahydrocannabinol (THC) and cannabidiol (CBD).[39] The primary cannabinoids, THC and CBD, are also the most abundant cannabis plant chemicals and are the cannabis components receiving the most attention from a medical perspective. While multiple other plant cannabinoids exist, including cannabinol (CBN), cannabigerol (CBG), and cannabichromene (CBC), that undoubtedly have therapeutic effects, evidence on specific use in human disease is currently limited and is beyond the scope of this text.

Most cannabinoids exist in the plant in acid form and are referred to with an attached letter *A*, such as THC-A and CBD-A. While having potential medicinal properties in their own right, the naturally occurring acid forms of plant cannabinoids are often thought to be inactive in humans. The active and more commonly known cannabinoids, including THC and CBD, are produced by decarboxylation via heat. Within the cannabis plant, most of the known cannabinoids are closely structurally related and are often precursors or derivatives of other cannabinoids along biosynthetic and breakdown pathways. In simple language, those pathways are processes where cannabinoid A may be broken down in the plant to form cannabinoids B and C, and these compounds may be used by the plant to produce cannabinoid D, and so forth. A similar process happens within our own bodies with hormones, neurotransmitters, and other compounds. Researchers are actively investigating the potential therapeutic benefits of the many lesser-known cannabinoids and their metabolic products.

Much of what we know about cannabinoids is the result of the research efforts of one man and his students. In 1964, Israeli scientist Raphael Mechoulam was looking for a novel area of study and realized that no one had determined what compounds were responsible for the reported effects of recreational cannabis. He had access to cannabis material that was being confiscated on the Lebanese border by Israeli police, and he obtained a few kilograms of hashish (concentrated cannabis resin). He used chromatography and analytical chemical extraction to obtain a series of reproducible compounds that he could reliably extract from the hashish samples. He then conducted experiments on animal and human test subjects to determine the effects of these compounds, discovering that only one of these extracted compounds was psychoactive. Further research elucidated the compound's chemical structure, and we now know this cannabinoid as delta9-tetrahydrocannabinol, usually just referred to as tetrahydrocannabinol or THC.

THC

Tetrahydrocannabinol is one of the primary cannabinoids, and it's the most predominant cannabinoid in most medical cannabis varietals. It's the only known cannabinoid compound that produces significant psychoactive effects, here meaning behavioural changes, impairment, or intoxication. Psychoactivity to the point of impairment is usually of no medical benefit and is normally considered an unwanted side effect of THC. However, by some definition, any compound that works on the central nervous system is psychoactive and this applies to all phytocannabinoids. THC just happens to be the only plant cannabinoid that is psychoactive to the point of altering normal function. Although most of the side effects and potential harms associated with cannabis use are attributed to THC, it is the best-researched cannabinoid and the chemical responsible for many of the cannabis plant's proven therapeutic benefits. THC has known benefits in the treatment of chronic neuropathic pain, pain and spasticity of multiple sclerosis, chemotherapy-induced nausea and vomiting, and anorexia and cachexia of HIV/AIDS. Emerging evidence also suggests benefit of THC in post-traumatic stress disorder (PTSD), insomnia, and other conditions.

THC appears to work primarily through direct effects on cannabinoid receptors in the central nervous system. Sought by recreational users as a "high," THC-associated psychoactive effects include euphoria, sedation, giddiness, increased appetite, and time distortion. High-dose THC products also pose increased risk of impairment, substance abuse, reduced cognitive functioning, and acute and chronic psychosis. However, when used in the lower doses typical of medical cannabis products, THC is very safe; I discuss the safety profile and potential side effects of cannabis medicine in detail in Chapter 5. Additionally, when used in conjunction with other cannabinoids, such as CBD, THC's side effects are lessened and its therapeutic benefits enhanced. Although not yet verified by strong data, CBD products also appear to work better when at least a small amount of THC is present.

This synergistic therapeutic enhancement is one reason many people believe that whole-plant cannabis medicine (discussed later in this chapter), or at least an extract containing multiple plant compounds, is better than single-cannabinoid cannabis medicine alone. Though researchers are trying to prove or disprove this theory, the cannabis plant is so complex and contains so many chemicals that years of research will be required to fully understand how phytocannabinoids work within the human body. Ultimately, so many variables are involved that scientific certainty will likely prove elusive for many years to come.

CBD

Cannabidiol is the second most abundant primary cannabinoid and is currently the subject of the most active medical interest. This interest comes from the fact that CBD seems to relieve many symptoms but does not cause impairment or intoxication. Additionally, CBD counteracts the side effects of THC without reducing its medical benefit. Therefore, using medicine that includes CBD (particularly for cannabis-naive patients who have no previous cannabis experience) is almost always recommended. CBD-predominant medicines are also recommended for patients who are trying to avoid side effects and patients wanting relief of symptoms without impairment. A recent polling of Canadian cannabis physicians revealed that the majority of their patients were requesting high-CBD or CBD-predominant* cannabis medicine.[40] Consequently, a lot of research is underway to determine which health conditions may benefit from CBD. Already, research published in 2017 verified the long-standing belief that CBD was anti-epileptic.[41] We also know that CBD is anti-inflammatory and an effective pain medicine for many patients with inflammatory-type pain. Additionally, it's an antioxidant and likely has neuroprotective properties.

As a further testament to its medical potential, based on research at the National Institutes of Health showing the potential neuroprotective properties of CBD, the US government was issued patent US6630507 in October 2003—despite the government's stance that cannabis has no known medical benefits. The issuance of this now-expired patent was a direct contradiction to the government's own classification of cannabis as a Schedule I drug. It represented the hypocrisy of simultaneously denying medicinal value while at the same time holding a patent based on known beneficial properties. However, in a sign of the dramatically changing times, the US DEA recently announced that it will consider rescheduling any CBD-based drugs approved by the US Food and Drug Administration (FDA), and the FDA recently approved a specific CBD cannabis extract, Epidiolex, for the treatment of drug-resistant pediatric epilepsy.

---

* High-CBD cannabis is a relative term and refers to cannabis products that contain high CBD content compared to the historical average for available strains, which was less than 1 percent CBD per dry weight. High-CBD strains currently available contain 10 to 20 percent CBD per dry weight. The term CBD-predominant refers to a strain where CBD is the predominat cannabinoid relative to THC. Cannabis strains currently on the market tend to fall into one of three categories related to the ratio of CBD to THC: CBD-predominant (relatively little THC), balanced CBD:THC, and THC-predominant (relatively little CBD). In this book, I use the the the terms according to these definitions, but note that it's possible to have a high-CBD strain (for example, 10 percent CBD per dry weight) that is also a THC-predominant strain if the percentage of THC is still significantly higher than the CBD percentage.

Terpenes

Terpenes, also sometimes referred to as terpenoids, are a large and common group of chemicals known as aromatic hydrocarbons. They are widely produced by many plants and even by some insects. They are the chemicals that make flowers smell like flowers, lemons smell like lemons, and pine needles smell like pine needles. They are commonly used to give aroma to perfumes and other beauty products. Terpenes often aid plants in attracting beneficial insects or repelling pests. They are also an important part of active plant metabolism and physiology. More than a dozen common terpenes are present in cannabis, but these compounds are not unique to cannabis and are also found in other plant species.

Terpenes are key components in essential oils, which are complex mixtures of volatile organic compounds that are vital in giving plants their characteristic aromas, flavours, and essences. For example, essential oil from lemons predominantly contains the terpene limonene. It's mostly limonene that gives lemons and other citrus fruits their distinct aroma. Essential oils have had reported health benefits for centuries, with many being known antioxidants and antiseptic agents. Due to their appealing aromas and reported medicinal benefits, they were often valued in ancient societies. Frankincense and myrrh, for instance, are essential oils that are heavy in terpenes and are featured in biblical stories. They were considered to be valuable as potential medicinal agents and were commonly traded in the ancient middle east.

While anecdotal evidence has suggested the benefits of essential oils for much of human history, so many terpenes exist in so many different plants that formal research into all of their specific benefits has not occurred until recently. Israel is now a leader in ongoing cannabis and terpene-specific research. However, the fact that terpenes are such widely abundant and common chemicals means that they can't be patented. This ubiquity limits their potential profitability and lessens the interest of any corporation to invest the huge amounts of money required to study new medicines. However, it may be possible to patent a novel proprietary blend of terpenes and cannabinoids that have a proven therapeutic effect. Hopefully, along with the current enthusiasm for cannabinoid research will come the desire to validate previously anecdotal claims of terpene benefits.

Despite a lack of scientific evidence, terpenes have become very popular in both the recreational and medical cannabis markets as consumers report very different effects depending on the terpene profile of the plant. Some early research data support the theory that phytocannabinoid–terpene interactions could produce additive effects when treating medical conditions.[42] For example, terpenes may help cannabinoids work better, and cannabinoids may similarly potentiate the therapeutic effects of terpenes. This synergy, known as the *entourage effect,* suggests that a mixture of cannabis chemicals together is more effective than the individual components alone (we'll explore this idea of the entourage effect and whole plant medicine in more detail later in the chapter). Varying terpene profiles are likely a major reason why different cannabis strains produce such different effects.[42]

Many producers are now trying to market and grow strains with distinct terpene profiles linked to specific therapeutic effects desired by patients and consumers. The most common terpenes in cannabis are myrcene, limonene, pinene, linalool, caryophyllene, nerolidol, phytol, terpineol, and borneol. Below I describe the top five common cannabis terpenes and their reported, albeit sometimes scientifically unproven, benefits and effects.

Myrcene

The most abundant terpene in cannabis, myrcene is known for its strong sedative and pain-reducing properties as well as for potentiating the effects of THC. It's a terpene associated with indica cannabis varietals known for producing a heavy relaxing and sedating effect. Patients who do not like, or are sensitive to, THC effects may not do well with high-myrcene strains. Myrcene is found in other plants, including thyme, basil, lemongrass, mango, and hops. Some recreational users reportedly eat mangoes to get more myrcene and strengthen the THC-driven cannabis high.

Limonene

The second most common cannabis terpene, limonene, is more widely associated with citrus fruits and gives these fruits their characteristic aromas. It's widely used in perfume and hand cleanser products, and its antimicrobial properties also make it a useful cleaning agent. Cannabis strains high in limonene are reported to be uplifting, euphoric, and anxiety relieving.

Pinene

This abundant terpene is well known to anyone who has walked through a pine tree forest or who has used the cleaning agent Pine-Sol. Pinene is one of the main components that gives pine needles their aroma. In the medical world, it's a known bronchodilator, which may explain why high-pinene strains reportedly relieve asthma. Pinene is also an antiseptic and possibly has anti-carcinogenic properties. In the cannabis world, it's known to counter the effects of THC and increase alertness.

Caryophyllene

This terpene is present in cloves and black pepper and, not surprisingly, has a peppery and spicy aroma. It has anti-inflammatory and analgesic properties and is known to reduce the anxiety and paranoia that a cannabis high sometimes produces. Experienced recreational users sometimes suggest chewing on black peppercorns or cloves if a cannabis high is too intense. Caryophyllene is one of the most powerful terpenes in cannabis, and since it appears to display some direct activation of cannabinoid receptors, some scientists think it might be considered a cannabinoid in its own right.

Linalool

This terpene is most closely associated with the aroma of lavender, the essential oil of which linalool is a major component. Just like the lavender plant, linalool is known as a calming and relaxing terpene. It's known to have anti-convulsant, anti-anxiety, anti-depressant, and potential anti-psychotic properties. People with mental illnesses have been observed to prefer and self-select high linalool strains.

Flavonoids

Like terpenes, flavonoids are not unique to cannabis plants and are found widely in many plant species. They are a large and complex group of chemicals that are metabolically active within plants. They are pigments and give fruits and vegetables their characteristic colours. They also have reported health benefits, including being powerful antioxidants. They are one of the reasons that deeply pigmented fruits and vegetables are reported to be so good for us. Also like terpenes, their use as medicine is not supported by any rigorous conventional medical research, likely due to the factors discussed in the terpene section above. It's highly likely, but scientifically unproven, that cannabis strains rich in antioxidant flavonoid compounds have additive therapeutic properties beyond just the cannabinoid and terpenoid content.

VARIETALS

As previously discussed, the cannabis plant has a number of varietals. Whether these forms represent different species, subspecies, or simply adaptive manifestations of one primary plant type is still up for debate. What matters to medical patients is that these differing forms of the cannabis plant tend to produce different mixtures of chemicals. A good example is the hemp varietal of cannabis, which typically produces very little THC. When medical cannabis is purchased as a purified extract of specific cannabinoids, the underlying plant varietal does not matter much. However, when using whole plant extracts or dried flower product, the varietal of origin may change the resulting mixture of plant chemicals more significantly. Ultimately, it's the mixture of chemicals that determines the effect rather than the name of a plant varietal or species. However, some of these traditional names persist and are worth discussing further in order to better understand medical cannabis.

Sativa versus Indica

One of the most dominant traditional cannabis classifications is between the sativa and indica varietals, also commonly referred to as strains. Experienced users of recreational cannabis often describe significant differences between the effects of sativa strains and indica strains. Typically, sativa strains reportedly produce an energetic or uplifting high while indica strains are usually associated with a more sedating and relaxing experience. In truth, most available cannabis strains today are a hybrid between these two main forms. Some evidence suggests that the majority of recreational psychoactive strains, typically high in THC, take their primary origin from indica varietals, whereas the genetics for medicinal strains, usually higher in CBD, tend to come from sativa varietals. Hemp varietals are also believed to be of sativa origin.

Regardless of classification disputes, many medical cannabis prescribers are steering away from making sativa or indica recommendations. Instead, they are primarily making recommendations based on the cannabinoid content of the strain in question, including the relative ratio of THC to CBD and other cannabinoids, and sometimes also to the terpene profile, if known. Ultimately, the chemical profile of the particular cannabis strain is what determines its effects rather than its underlying lineage. This chemical composition is determined by many factors, including soil composition, light spectrum, and presence or absence of predators or disease. In the future, medical cannabis will likely be sold based on known chemical composition rather than on the sativa versus indica differentiation.

Cannabis versus Hemp

At the most basic level, hemp is just a type of cannabis with a very low concentration of psychoactive and medicinal chemicals. The differences in chemical production are due to adaptations of different varietals within the same cannabis family. These variations get back to the previous sativa versus indica discussion. Regardless of whether they are separate species or just variants of one species, sativa plants tend to be more fibre rich with longer and thicker stems, whereas indica plants tend to be bushier and produce more concentrated cannabinoids in the resin of their flowers. Therefore, the hemp varietal of cannabis is primarily from sativa heritage. This varietal can grow very tall, and plants up to 6 m (20 ft) are not uncommon. Plants grown for their concentrated medicinal chemicals tend to be much shorter, 1 to 2 m (3 to 6 ft). Hemp varietals of cannabis are typically grown to produce fibre and seeds, whereas medical and recreational cannabis varietals are grown to produce the concentrated plant chemicals we know as cannabinoids.

Because hemp and medical cannabis have different growing characteristics and are grown for different reasons, they require different growing conditions and produce different levels of active chemicals. In hemp production, both female and male plants are allowed to survive and pollinate to produce seeds and the next generation. With medical cannabis, only female plants are emphasized since they produce the concentrated medicinal chemicals. While the differences in morphology (the appearance of the plant) and growing conditions help differentiate the varietals, it's the variance in THC content that produces the primary distinction in terms of both classification and regulation. Hemp is defined as cannabis that has a maximum THC content of 0.3 percent. In contrast, medical and recreational cannabis plants may have up to 30 percent THC content. Because hemp plants produce so little THC, their production has not been regulated in the same way as production of other cannabis plants has. This situation is somewhat confusing since in most ways they are the same plant. This separate regulation of hemp has resulted in widespread marketing and sale of hemp-derived CBD in some jurisdictions where low-THC/high-CBD extract from another form of cannabis is illegal.

The fact that hemp is regulated separately from other cannabis varietals leads to an obvious question: what is the difference between THC or CBD obtained from hemp versus that obtained from medical cannabis plants? The easy answer is that there is no difference on a molecular basis. Both hemp and cannabis are varietals of the same plant, and a molecule of pure THC or CBD from a hemp plant is therefore identical to a molecule of pure THC or CBD from another cannabis plant. Medical and recreational varietal cannabis tends to produce more THC, and hemp varietal cannabis tends to produce more CBD and very little THC, but both compounds are the same in each case.

Even though a molecule of THC or CBD from a hemp plant is identical to the same chemicals from a medical plant, the extracts from hemp and medical cannabis plants often differ based on the total concentration of other plant chemicals and cannabinoids. Hemp always contains less THC, and often less of some other active plant chemicals, than medical cannabis. However, it often contains relatively more CBD, and some hemp varietals may also have a wide spectrum of other cannabinoids. Therefore, hemp extracts may or may not contain fewer cannabinoids or a lower spectrum of additional active chemicals, such as terpenes, than would occur with a medical cannabis plant extract. Most important is the fact that the hemp extract market is largely unregulated, and the products have traditionally been treated as health supplements. The source and composition of hemp extracts, therefore, are often unknown and of dubious quality, composition, and purity. While there is currently a resurgence in the Canadian and US hemp industries, many hemp-based products on the North American market were previously shipped in from overseas without any regulation, and it was unclear what was in those products. While the lack of consistency and quality of available hemp products may change with future regulations, currently the best source of medical cannabis extracts are from regulated Canadian LPs.

WHOLE PLANT MEDICINE

Within the cannabis plant are hundreds of chemical compounds, including the already-mentioned phytocannabinoids, terpenes, and flavonoids. The potential additive effect of this entire group of chemicals working together to give full medical benefit is called the *entourage effect*, which is a tenet of whole plant medicine. This concept suggests that taking medicine from the whole plant is better than taking isolated cannabinoids. While many cannabis advocates and long-time users claim that cannabis compounds act in concert to give a combined effect, most available research has been done on cannabis strains with unknown chemical compositions or on THC and CBD alone. Therefore, we currently have little data specifically supporting the entourage effect and the idea that medicating with the whole cannabis plant is significantly better than using individual cannabinoid preparations. We do, however, know that the combination of THC and CBD seems to be more effective than either cannabinoid alone, but even that relationship has not been well studied. We also know that cannabis strains with different terpene profiles have very different user-reported effects. We just lack conclusive data supporting the entourage effect theory.

Despite this lack of evidence, some North American producers have started to create cannabis products with set mixtures and concentrations of cannabinoids and terpenes designed to produce specific effects. They sell these products as proprietary blends, mostly in US states where cannabis is legal, often labelled for the desired outcome. Examples of such product names are Bliss, Relief, Calm, Passion, and Arouse. There is no conclusive evidence that these special blends work, but ongoing scientific studies are attempting to match certain cannabinoid/terpenoid/flavonoid profiles to specific therapeutic effects. The challenge of this research is that with every added variable, definitive scientific conclusions (on a statistical basis) become much harder to reach. Some scientists say that beyond four or five variables reasonable certainty is not possible. That limitation makes definitive answers regarding the entourage effect extremely difficult or impossible.

The entourage effect is, therefore, both a blessing and a curse: it's a blessing that the remarkable cannabis plant contains so many therapeutically active compounds, but it's a curse for scientists trying to answer basic cannabis questions. There are simply too many variables. This problem contributes to the polarization of those for and against cannabis. Though much loved by the recreational users and medical cannabis evangelists, the entourage effect is not endorsed by many conventional health care providers who were trained on the single molecule–single disease pharmaceutical model. To them, the concept is too loose and too unscientific. Years of additional research are needed to bridge this gap. Luckily, that research is underway, and some labs have started the slow and potentially painstaking process of evaluating the possible therapeutic benefit of increasingly complex mixtures of cannabis chemicals.

ACCESSING MEDICINAL PROPERTIES
As discussed, the most potent medically active chemicals in cannabis are found in the resin produced by the trichome glands in the flowers

of the female cannabis plant. Any effective method of concentrating, activating, and ingesting these compounds can be used to access the medicinal properties of the plant. Traditional methods of producing concentrated cannabis products involved collecting loose trichome resin glands into a powder, known as kief, or compressing the resin into a form known as hashish. Extracts can also be made by using alcohol or oils to extract cannabinoids, since these compounds are fat soluble and won't dissolve in water. Unfortunately, most of these methods are laborious, time consuming, and relatively unrefined for a modern medical patient.

The primary traditional method of using medical cannabis was through inhalation of smoke produced by burning the dried buds of the female cannabis flower, a method currently not recommended due to potential smoking-related health risks. Alternatively, the extracts or concentrates mentioned above could be made and either ingested orally or burned and inhaled. These limited options for accessing the medically active compounds in cannabis led to the current push to find and develop more refined and accurate delivery methods, which I discuss in Chapter 11. In the next section, I review how medical cannabis chemicals are activated and introduce the products currently available to medical cannabis patients in Canada.

Activating Medicinal Components

In the raw cannabis plant, the cannabinoid compounds exist mostly in acid form. Chemically speaking, being in acid form means that the compounds contain something called a carboxyl group (COOH). The carboxyl group makes most cannabinoid acids inactive in the human body, and the cannabinoids must be decarboxylated by heat in order to become therapeutically active. Decarboxylation removes the attached carboxyl group, allowing the remaining cannabinoid molecules to activate the cannabinoid receptors in the human body.

The primary required components of decarboxylation are heat and time, with higher temperatures causing faster decarboxylation. While some partial decarboxylation occurs while drying and curing cannabis flower at room temperature, decarboxylation occurs almost instantly when the temperature is over 200°C (400°F), as with the heat of smoking or high-temperature vaporizing. While smoking involves burning by combustion at temperatures 300 to 550°C (600 to 1000°F), a more controlled release of cannabinoids may be obtained by vaporizing at lower temperatures since each cannabinoid decarboxylates at a slightly different temperature.

Heat decarboxylation of most cannabinoids begins at approximately 100°C (215°F), but full decarboxylation at this temperature may take more than forty-five minutes. This slower approach to decarboxylation is used when making edible cannabis products. For use in edibles, cannabis needs to be heated at a lower temperature over a longer period of time to decarboxylate the cannabinoids slowly while avoiding burning or vaporizing off the medicinal components. To preserve the cannabinoids, heat must be kept below approximately 175°C (350°F). Though a thorough discussion of decarboxylation temperatures is beyond the scope of this book, interested readers can find more information online and directly from many LPs.

There are proponents of ingesting raw, un-decarboxylated cannabis, but scientific evidence supporting health benefits is lacking. The story of someone becoming instantly dysfunctional and inebriated after eating raw cannabis is mostly fictional, although there are some effects. As explained Part I, ancient people likely discovered the medicinal and psychoactive properties of cannabis by eating plant parts. This discovery can be explained by the fact that some decarboxylation occurs in the body after eating raw cannabis, and some decarboxylation occurs with drying and time, though much less than occurs with higher-temperature heating. Even though emerging evidence suggests some potential medical benefits of eating or juicing raw cannabis, only by decarboxylating can most of the known important medical cannabinoid molecules have full therapeutic effect.

As mentioned briefly above, a final consideration for activating cannabis medicine for use in edibles involves the fact that cannabis plant compounds are fat soluble and do not dissolve in water. They can be dissolved in oil, butter, alcohol, and other edible fats, like lard. Therefore, in order to efficiently extract the active medicinal cannabis compounds from whole plant material for use in edibles, a non-water-based extraction method is needed.

Available Medical Cannabis Products

Currently, the only legal medical products available to Canadian patients are sold through LPs and are varieties of dried cannabis flower and edible oil concentrates in liquid or gelcap form. As pharmacies start to enter the legal medical cannabis market, a wider variety of medical cannabis products are likely to become available, including topicals, tablets, nebulizers, and transdermal patches. The government has stated that under the new Cannabis Act cannabis edibles won't be available for at least a year after recreational legalization, and it's unclear if they will ever be available in the separate medical stream. Edibles are defined as cannabis-infused food or beverage products and are not currently available from any LP as they weren't sanctioned under the original ACMPR. Health Canada's reluctance to offer edibles as medicine through LPs may stem from the fact that dosing with edibles is difficult to control, and the products often look like desirable treats. The risk of children encountering adverse effects by ingesting too much cannabis via edibles is high. As the adult recreational cannabis market develops, it appears certain that edibles will eventually become widely available. The current investment into the cannabis industry by large beverage companies is testament to this fact. The majority of these products will likely be kept in the recreational category as oral formulations of cannabis medicine will certainly evolve to match other conventional pharmaceuticals.

Recreational cannabis concentrates, such as shatter (a potent form of high-THC cannabis extract), are not available from LPs due to safety concerns since most theoretical harms of cannabis increase with the higher percentage of THC found in these products. Cannabis concentrates are more typically desired by a recreational market, and the potency of THC can reach 100 percent, which is not a product with significant medical benefit or need. The majority of medical cannabis products contain 20 percent or less THC whereas the majority of concentrates contain between 40 and 80 percent THC. Shatter, a particularly potent concentrate, usually contains 70 to 90 percent THC and has little theoretical benefit to medical consumers. As with edibles, it can be difficult to know how much cannabinoid is consumed when using potent concentrates. The result can be a prolonged and uncomfortable experience, which is opposite to the relief of symptoms without impairment intended by medical practitioners and patients.

CHAPTER 5
CANNABIS AND THE BODY

Only in the last few decades have we begun to discover how cannabis works in our bodies. Despite not previously understanding how cannabis exerted its effects, people chose to self-medicate with cannabis for relief of a multitude of symptoms. Even today, despite many advances, we have conclusive scientific evidence of medical cannabis benefit for only a limited number of conditions. These conditions include chronic neuropathic pain, chemotherapy-induced nausea and vomiting, and pain and spasticity of multiple sclerosis. Evidence is also strong for treatment of anorexia and cachexia of HIV/AIDS, drug-resistant pediatric epilepsy, and pain and suffering of palliative and oncology patients. A lack of evidence doesn't mean cannabis doesn't work for other conditions, it just means we don't have established scientific proof. In fact, the growing reports on ways cannabis can improve multiple diseases and symptoms—pain, appetite, nausea, spasticity, headaches, anxiety, Parkinson's, immune function, memory, seizures—can be overwhelming and stretch belief that any one medicine could possibly have so many uses. It doesn't really make sense and is usually not the case with pharmaceuticals, which are typically targeted to one symptom or disease process.

Why is cannabis different? The answer lies in the fact that cannabis is not one drug. Rather, it's a plant that contains multiple medicines. These multiple compounds exert a variety of effects on an extensive network of receptors across many body systems. Despite the fact that we've now identified a plausible and increasingly understood mechanism by which cannabis works in the human body, it's important to realize that there is no miracle drug and that cannabis is no exception to this rule. It doesn't cure all diseases or assist with every ailment, but its astonishing range of efficacy across so many conditions is remarkable. In this chapter, I explore how this breadth of efficacy is possible. I review cannabis's safety profile, discuss how it functions in the human body, and discover how it may affect patients and behave under different conditions.

SAFETY PROFILE

Even before we understood how cannabis worked, we knew it had a remarkable and unparalleled track record of safety. Voluntary users of both recreational and medicinal products accept the risk of taking compounds into their bodies every day. In fact, many of the common medications and other substances humans choose to ingest have significant risks. Coffee, for example, has over twenty-five serious potential interactions with prescription medications listed while cannabis has almost none. Approximately 450 people die every year in North America from acetaminophen overdose, and nonsteroidal anti-inflammatory drugs (NSAIDS), like ibuprofen, kill more than 16,000 people per year. Even water, natural and pure, can cause intoxication deaths and regularly does in North America. There are caffeine overdose deaths, and there have been deaths from ingestion of too much table salt. But surprisingly, there has never been a verified cannabis overdose death.

The only reported human deaths from cannabis are due to ingestion of heavily contaminated street product, product deliberately mixed with other narcotics, or synthetic cannabis analogue products, such as K2 or Spice. In primate animal studies, the LD-50 (the experimental dose of a drug at which 50 percent of test subjects die) of oral cannabis could not be calculated because none of the test subjects died.[43] Indeed, after receiving up to 9 g/kg oral THC (reportedly 150,000 times the minimal starting dose), test subject monkeys became somnolent and unresponsive for many hours but returned to normal health after the effects wore off. Due to lack of confirmatory evidence, the possible lethal dose of cannabis in humans is therefore only estimated. By some calculations, it would require ingestion of more than a thousand pounds of cannabis. By this estimate, a heavy bale of cannabis would only kill you if it fell on you and crushed you!

So why is cannabis so safe? Most street drugs, and even many medicines, are predictably deadly when taken in high doses. The explanation is that for most drugs, overdose deaths are cardiopulmonary, particularly due to suppression of respiratory drive and lack of airway protection. Basically, people stop breathing. Cannabis, however, does not interfere with breathing or suppress respiration. This attribute is likely the primary reason that cannabis overdose is unpleasant but not particularly dangerous.

Possible exceptions to the general rule that cannabis intoxication, most often the result of THC, is not particularly dangerous include severely impaired motor coordination, severe acute hyperemesis, severe acute cannabis psychosis causing increased risk of harm to self or others, and exacerbation of existing cardiac disease. Despite these risks, which I discuss in detail later in this chapter, the vast majority of cannabis studies have shown no major morbidity or mortality. A review of over three hundred cannabis studies showed that 97 percent of reported side effects were not serious.[44] No one has ever died from cannabis overdose, and on a daily basis, we accept much greater risks using common over-the-counter cold and pain medicines. The incredible safety profile of cannabis is one of the main reasons I am such a strong supporter of this natural medicine. Helping people without hurting them is the top goal of most health care providers. With cannabis medicine, that outcome is usually possible.

This unparalleled and almost unbelievable safety profile is one of the most remarkable things about cannabis. It's worth stating again: there have been no verified cannabis overdose deaths. This fact alone is truly remarkable. However, as already mentioned, this high level of safety does not mean cannabis is risk free, as there are no risk-free medicines. All medicines have side effects, including cannabis medicine, but life-threatening side effects are exceedingly rare with cannabis. This unmatched safety is likely one of the reasons cannabis was used medicinally for thousands of years in cultures around the world. People discovered that they could relieve symptoms without risking serious side effects or death.

THE ENDOCANNABINOID SYSTEM

The therapeutic effects of cannabis are mediated by a system in our bodies called the *endocannabinoid system* or *ECS*. This important biological system was discovered only recently, in 1992, as a direct result of Dr. Mechoulam's pioneering cannabis research. Despite more than five thousand scientific publications outlining the structure, function, and role of the ECS, this important component of human health has yet to be widely taught in medical schools. The system is remarkably complex, and even a superficial discussion involves technical and scientific vocabulary. For interested readers, the following paragraphs delve a little further into the ECS. For a more comprehensive understanding, readers may wish to explore the many basic science papers on the ECS that are available online.

Discovery and Research

We previously assumed that the human body must contain receptors that the phytocannabinoids interacted with to produce psychoactive and therapeutic effects, but their presence was only proven definitively in 1988. The existence of an internal biological system that produces cannabinoid molecules (the ECS) was then soon confirmed when researchers discovered a cannabis-like molecule, called *anandamide*, in 1992. Because anandamide was being produced internally, therefore classified as an *endo*cannabinoid, and was binding to our cannabinoid receptors, scientists could be sure that a human cannabinoid system existed.

The ECS is made up of three components—endocannabinoids, their associated receptors, and enzymes that aid in either generating or metabolizing those molecules—and functions independently of the cannabis plant in the same way that our endogenous opioid system functions independently of the opium poppy. In both cases, the human systems were named after the plants whose active molecules were discovered first. In our endogenous opioid system, our bodies produce endorphins that act like opium. In the ECS, our bodies produce endocannabinoids, like anandamide, that act like plant cannabinoids on our natural receptors. The ECS functions similarly to how neurotransmitter and cell-signalling mechanisms work within other better-known body systems, such as the nervous or digestive systems. We have also discovered that the ECS is found not only in humans but also in all vertebrates and many invertebrates as well.

However, despite nearly thirty years of active science investigating the ECS since anandamide's discovery, the system appears to be so widespread and complex that many questions remain unanswered. The ECS is not widely known or understood not only because it was discovered relatively recently, but also because its components can't be seen with the naked eye. It's much easier to understand and study, say, the digestive system, where you can see the stomach and intestines, or the cardiac system, where you can see the heart and blood vessels. The ECS, in contrast, is hidden from direct observation. These challenges aside, we have now gained a fundamental preliminary understanding of the ECS's components, the way phytocannabinoids interact with the ECS, and the role the ECS plays within the human body. Let's take a closer look at this fascinating system.

Endocannabinoids

The primary endocannabinoids are anandamide (2-arachidonoyl-ethanolamine) and 2-AG (2-arachidonoyl-glycerol), and they are produced on demand by the body from cell membrane phospholipids. Other cannabinoid-like compounds produced by our bodies that likely act on the ECS receptors include 2-arachidonoyl-glycerol-ether and N-arachidonoyl-dopamine. The endocannabinoids may be classified as neurotransmitters, neuromodulators, or neuro-immunomodulators, depending on how and where they are functioning in our bodies. They sometimes function like neurotransmitters to directly send neural signals, but more often they function like neuromodulators or neuro-immunomodulators. In those roles, they modulate, or adjust, the effects of other neurotransmitters and cell-signalling pathways throughout the body.

While research on these compounds is in its very early stages, we do know a little about how the endocannabinoids function. Though many neurotransmitters send direct forward messages down nerves, endocannabinoids, when functioning as neurotransmitters, appear to have a much more complex role. Research suggests that endocannabinoids work primarily in a retrograde fashion, sending chemical messages backward across neural junctions (synapses). A simple analogy would be like a train conductor sending messages from a downstream junction to influence train movement back at the home station. Additionally, it appears that rather than just sending backwards, or retrograde, neurotransmitter-like signals, the endocannabinoids also act as neuromodulators. In this role, they seem to exert and influence the function and behaviour of other existing neurotransmitter systems using complex mechanisms. When endocannabinoids activate cannabinoid receptors, which I discuss next, they often alter the flow of other neurotransmitters, such as serotonin, dopamine, and glutamate.

The endocannabinoids produce various effects within the human body, which we are only beginning to understand. Anandamide produces many pleasant effects and was given a Sanskrit name for joy and happiness. Due to this association, it's also sometimes referred to as "the bliss molecule." Animal studies have taught us that anandamide can also increase appetite and enhance pleasure associated with food consumption, and it's likely responsible for some of the rewarding effects of exercise (for example, the "runner's high"). Anandamide also appears to play a role in memory, motivation, sense of time, and pain perception. The role of 2-AG is not as well defined, but it appears to be predominantly related to inflammatory and immune functions. Evidence strongly suggests that there are more endocannabinoid molecules to be discovered.

Receptors

In order to function within the body, the endocannabinoid molecules require receptors with which to interact. These receptor molecules are the ECS components that facilitate the cannabinoid effects. Two primary cannabinoid receptors have been discovered, named CB1 and CB2. Both are found throughout the body but are most common in the brain and immune system. CB1 receptors are located primarily in the central and peripheral nervous systems whereas CB2 receptors are distributed primarily in peripheral organ and immune tissues. Researchers Devane and Howlett discovered the CB1 receptor in a rat brain at the Saint Louis University School of Medicine in Missouri in 1988,[45] a few years before discovery and evidence of the whole ECS system. We now know that CB1 receptors are found extensively in the brains of most mammals. By some estimates, there are more endocannabinoid receptors in the brain than any other specific neurotransmitter receptor, although this fact remains unverified. The CB2 receptor was discovered a few years later in 1993 by researchers Munro, Thomas, and Abu-Shaar at the MRC Laboratory of Molecular Biology in Cambridge, England.[46] Being primarily associated with the immune system, CB2 receptors are typically found outside of the brain in such places as the gut, spleen, liver, heart, kidneys, bones, blood vessels, lymph cells, endocrine glands, and reproductive organs.

Both CB1 and CB2 receptors are G protein coupled. G proteins, technically called *guanine-nucleotide binding proteins*, are a common family of protein molecules in our bodies, and G protein–coupled receptors are a large family of cell receptors that detect molecules outside cells and trigger resulting responses inside cells. G protein–coupled receptors are the most common form of cell-surface receptors that transmit messages across cell membranes. When a molecule outside the cell interacts with a matching receptor, the receptor initiates physiological responses within the cell. The propensity of a molecule to bind with a receptor is called *binding affinity*, which you can think of like electrical plug connecting to a wall socket. When a molecule, like a cannabinoid, "plugs" into a receptor "socket," it activates the receptor, which goes on to elicit a cellular response. This explanation is tidy and simplistic, but it turns out that the function of the endocannabinoids is more complex and mechanisms are often indirect. However, this analogy is useful for understanding the basic mechanisms of molecule-receptor interactions, and I use it throughout to help explain cannabinoid-receptor interactions. Ultimately, either through direct or indirect signalling mechanisms, the endocannabinoids produce their physiological effects, the diversity of which suggests the presence of not only additional cannabinoids but also undiscovered cannabinoid receptors and unexplained mechanisms.

Phytocannabinoids and the ECS

As discussed, phytocannabinoids are similar in structure to endocannabinoids and can therefore also function within the ECS by binding to and interacting with receptors. The different effects produced by the phytocannabinoids CBD and THC, reviewed in Chapter 4, are likely due to small differences in the molecular structures of the compounds. Their structures determine how each interacts with the different receptors. Since the CB1 receptors are concentrated in the brain and the central nervous system, interactions with those receptors are most likely to produce psychoactive effects. So when considering the psychoactive effects of cannabis, we're primarily dealing with how the phytocannabinoids interact with the CB1 receptors.

THC has high binding affinity for CB1 receptors while CBD has low binding affinity, which likely explains why THC produces psychoactive effects while CBD does not. Returning to our plug-and-socket analogy, a THC plug is shaped to connect with CB1 sockets. When that connection happens, THC activates those CB1 receptors. Researchers therefore call THC a CB1 receptor *agonist*. THC mimics anandamide, which also directly activates CB1 receptors. THC's plug resembles anandamide closely enough that it's able to influence the CB1 receptor directly, allowing it to produce some of the same blissful feelings. THC is also the compound that causes most of the potential side effects of cannabis, particularly when taken in doses that greatly exceed any potential effect of the naturally produced anandamide. This effect is similar to the situation with opioids, where endogenous opioids would never stop a person from breathing whereas heroin easily can. Same receptors, but different effects due to dosing and potency.

CBD, by contrast, is not a particularly good fit with CB1 receptors, and the mechanisms by which it interacts with the CB1 receptor are poorly understood. We know that it primarily acts as an *antagonist* of direct CB1 agonists, like THC and anandamide, although it can have variable agonistic or antagonistic effects on other neurotransmitters. In other words, CBD does not appear to directly activate or suppress CB1 receptors. Rather, it suppresses the CB1-activating qualities of a cannabinoid like THC. Therefore, CBD tends to oppose the action of THC at the CB1 receptor, thus muting the psychoactive effects of THC. This modulating effect of CBD is why patients may have fewer THC-related side effects if they take a balanced dose of CBD with THC. Interestingly though, CBD does not seem to interfere with the medical benefits of THC, possibly because those effects require only very minimal THC-receptor activation.

The exact mechanisms by which CBD works are still poorly understood. Interestingly, its endocannabinoid analog, 2-AG, also works through mechanisms that are not well defined. Both 2-AG and CBD seem to work in complex and often indirect ways on both the CB1 and CB2 receptors. Overall, CBD tends to be a better fit to CB2 receptors than CB1 receptors but also seems to influence CB2 receptors in a more indirect way than the "plug-in-socket" fashion of THC and CB1. Until recently, researchers believed that CB2 receptors played no obvious direct role in nerve signalling and had little role in brain function. However, studies now verify that CB2 receptors play an important, yet poorly understood, role in the signal processing of the brain and peripheral tissues.

Function

Evidence suggests that the ECS regulates homeostasis, or balance, processes within our bodies. This regulation occurs in areas as diffuse as appetite, inflammation, pain perception, mood, and memory. Increasing evidence suggests that when the ECS is not working properly, physical symptoms and illness may result. This idea, first postulated by research scientist Ethan Russo in 2004,[47] supports the notion that cannabis medicine works by mimicking the body's natural endocannabinoids. By improving or restoring function to the ECS, medical cannabis relieves symptoms and possibly even resolves the underlying illness. Theoretically, problems with the ECS could develop due to deficiency or excess of receptors, deficiency or excess of endocannabinoids, or dysfunction of the signalling process, including defects in related enzyme function. All of these areas are actively being investigated, and much attention is being paid to developing cannabinoid medicines that will target specific cell-signalling pathways within the ECS.

The ECS is fundamental, widespread, and incredibly complex. While we still have more unanswered questions than known facts, it's fascinating to consider that the ECS is widely established in nature throughout all vertebrates and many invertebrate species. Research and discovery into the role of the ECS in other animals may help us understand why we contain the same system. We have discovered that the ECS has multiple roles in invertebrate physiology, including regulation of sensation, reproduction, feeding behaviour, neurotransmission, and inflammation. This system appears to be so fundamental and important that it was widely preserved and retained during evolution. That fact suggests that with further research into the ECS and cannabis medicine, we may be on the verge of important discoveries related to human health and disease, in areas from neurodegenerative disorders to inflammatory bowel disease. The fundamental importance and diffuse nature of the ECS help to explain why the cannabis plant and its phytocannabinoids have such a remarkably broad range of effects. Through direct interaction with our bodies' own ECS, cannabis medicine is able to provide treatment and relief of an extraordinary range of symptoms and diseases.

SIDE EFFECTS AND POTENTIAL HARMS

Because Canada is the first large Western democracy to federally legalize cannabis, much of the world will be watching and looking for answers to a number of questions regarding the drug's potential harms, both on individuals and on the entire population: What are the widespread behavioural, social, and economic consequences of federal legalization? What are the long-term community health outcomes associated with widespread public use? Will legalization affect use patterns in teens and children? Health Canada and the provincial health ministries are appropriately emphasizing a harm-reduction approach and have been gathering data from the outset. The data we have from US states that have legalized cannabis suggest that many projected potential harms have not been demonstrated. Some potential harms, like driving risk, are still being observed and monitored. Issues of community and public health will remain paramount as Canada leads the democratic world in reversing almost a century of cannabis prohibition.

It's important to realize that almost all of our data regarding risks of cannabis come from studies on the effects of smoked recreational product. Therefore, until we get data on specific medical formulations and products, potential risks of medical cannabis will have to be inferred from those prior studies. No pharmacological agent is free from potential toxicity and side effects, and medical cannabis is no exception. While there have been no verified deaths due to cannabis overdose, the acute (early) and chronic (long-term) side effects discussed herein warrant a careful approach by both patients and providers.

Acute Side Effects

Almost all acute side effects are the result of temporary THC intoxication after use of high-THC recreational products. Potentially dangerous acute adverse effects include severe nausea and vomiting (hyperemesis), paranoia and anxiety, suicidal ideations and tendencies, psychotic symptoms, and significantly impaired coordination and motor control. Though this impairment is rarely dangerous itself, cannabis intoxication is associated with an increased risk of motor vehicle accidents, which obviously has the potential of serious injury and mortality.

While cannabis medicine is often effective in treating nausea and vomiting, cannabis use is paradoxically also associated with both an acute and a chronic form of hyperemesis, the latter of which I discuss in the next section. Acute hyperemesis occurs in less than 5 percent of users, typically younger, cannabis-naive users exposed to cannabis for the first time. The problem usually goes away rapidly on its own but is very unpleasant and could be dangerous in rare cases due to dehydration or injuries to the GI tract from severe repetitive vomiting. Cases that persist beyond a few hours may need assessment and intravenous rehydration in the ER.

Cannabis has many additional potential acute side effects, most of which aren't dangerous, including euphoria, altered mood, impaired cognition, red eyes, dry mouth, increased appetite, dizziness, coughing, drowsiness or sedation, nausea, vomiting, increased heart rate, increase or decrease in blood pressure, anxiety, paranoia, and panic attacks. Some reported effects, like coughing, are mostly the result of smoking, which is not recommended for medicinal use.

The goal of medical cannabis treatment is to relieve symptoms without causing side effects, and most low-THC or non-THC medical products cause significantly fewer acute side effects than high-THC recreational products. However, even with medical products, experiencing some side effects is still possible. Many of the potentially desirable and pleasant effects of cannabis for recreational users may be experienced as unpleasant or negative by users who are naive to cannabis or who are particularly sensitive to the effects of THC. The psychoactive cannabis effects that produce pleasant euphoria for some users may be experienced as anxiety or paranoia in others. Among the most common potential side effects of cannabis medicine, acute impairment of coordination and motor performance is also likely the most dangerous. A strong recommendation not to operate machinery or drive a vehicle while impaired, or with risk of impairment on a new medication, must be followed. Temporary impairment of short-term memory and cognitive processing also means strict avoidance of situations where one requires sharpness and full control.

I must stress again that most cannabis side effects appear to be THC related, and these THC effects can usually be mitigated in medical patients by lowering THC dosage and/or taking a balanced dose of CBD. As mentioned previously, CBD tends to reduce the unpleasant side effects of THC. Pure-THC side effects range from pleasant or neutral through mildly unpleasant, up to severe and incapacitating. No matter what a patient's subjective experience, however, it's important to remember that acute side effects are transient, self-limited (meaning they go away on their own), and almost never dangerous. Patients with significant THC toxicity may feel as if they are about to die, but they are not. To many people, this idea makes no sense, but as already discussed, cannabis has an unmatched safety profile and no overdose deaths have ever been reported.

Chronic Side Effects

What potential long-term cannabis harms do we know about? Surprisingly, it has been hard to verify or prove that cannabis causes any common well-defined harms despite long-term use. However, we do know of some potential chronic side effects, which are associated primarily with high-THC cannabis. Potential chronic adverse effects include cannabinoid hyperemesis syndrome, exacerbation or unmasking of psychotic disorders (particularly in genetically susceptible people), cannabis use disorder, increased risk of mood disorders, withdrawal symptoms, neurocognitive impairment, and increased risk of cardiovascular and respiratory disease. Frequent and prolonged use of cannabis may also be associated with deterioration of both mental and physical health.

Cannabinoid Hyperemesis Syndrome

Chronic hyperemesis associated with cannabis use is rare, but the condition is currently receiving a lot of attention. An increasingly recognized syndrome of cyclical vomiting and abdominal pain in the setting of chronic cannabis use is known as cannabinoid hyperemesis syndrome (CHS). Patients often have low-grade nausea and abdominal pain with recurrent intermittent episodes of more severe vomiting. Dehydration, weight loss, and mild nutritional deficits are common during periods of increased vomiting, but patients may return to mostly normal health during occasional symptom-free periods.[48] Emergency room visits for this syndrome have reportedly increased in most jurisdictions in which cannabis legalization has occurred.[49]

CHS is associated with heavy long-term recreational cannabis use,[50] and there is no data to suggest such an association with use of lower-THC medical products. Often, years of recreational cannabis use precede development of CHS.[51] The condition was not commonly associated with recreational cannabis use in the past. Since this syndrome has become increasingly recognized over the last few years, some have suggested that its prevalence is a consequence of more widespread use of higher-THC recreational products that have be-come available only recently.[52]

The cause of CHS is not known but is likely related to the paradox-ical effects of THC taken in excess doses that I discussed previously. This paradoxical effect explains why intermittent use of low-dose medical cannabis is effective at treating nausea and vomiting, while frequent use of high-dose recreational product can produce opposite effects. Excess cannabis use may disrupt the balance of the ECS, resulting in dysregulation of the endogenous cannabinoids and asso-ciated cannabinoid receptors. Research has shown that cannabis may slow gastrointestinal (GI) motility, particularly if used chronically, and this reduced motility may precipitate hyperemesis. CHS appears clinically similar to cyclical vomiting syndrome (CVS), which is a condition of recurrent vomiting that occurs without cannabis use. Both CVS and CHS likely have components of reduced GI motility as an underlying cause of the GI symptoms. Patients with CHS are often diagnosed with CVS until the underlying chronic cannabis use is discovered.[53]

Treatment for chronic hyperemesis is divided into two phases: the first is initial supportive therapy to control the active symptoms, and the second is an ongoing treatment plan to help prevent recurrence and relapse. Initial supportive therapy addresses rehydration and nutritional support to counter the fluid, electrolyte, and nutritional losses of persistent recurrent vomiting. For unknown reasons, pa-tients with CHS tend to get the most relief of symptoms from frequent hot baths or showers, and history of very frequent bathing is often present.[50] The only known permanent treatment for CHS is cannabis cessation. The ongoing treatment and relapse prevention phase usual-ly involves substance abuse counselling and support as CHS is often part of a larger problem of cannabis use disorder. The CHS relapse rate of patients who continue with smoked recreational cannabis use is high. There haven't been any reports of CHS after exclusive use of cannabis edibles or other non-inhaled cannabis products. We cur-rently lack data to show whether patients with a prior history of CHS would tolerate or be appropriate candidates for specific medical can-nabis products once they have stopped recreational use.

Psychotic Disorders

The connection between cannabis and psychotic disorders is likely the most well-known and most concerning potential chronic side effect of cannabis use, though the exact risks are hard to define. We know that high-dose THC can cause acute psychosis in recreational users and that the risk increases with higher potency and synthetic cannabis products. We also know fairly definitively that cannabis can cause an earlier onset of chronic psychosis in genetically vulnerable patients. What is unclear is the extent to which, if any, cannabis contributes to the development of psychotic illness in individuals who are not already predisposed to psychosis.

If cannabis was an obvious contributor to the development of schizophrenia or other psychotic illness, we would expect to see a much higher incidence of these diseases in populations with high cannabis use. That situation does not appear to be the case. However, enough epidemiologic evidence links cannabis use to some small, as yet undefined, increased risk of psychotic illness that a consensus is that cannabis use should be avoided by children and teenagers since their brains are still developing. This concern is particularly relevant for children with a family history of psychotic mental illness. In the case of specific use of medical cannabis products, we have no evidence that non-THC or low-THC medical products increase psychotic risk at all. However, the consensus remains that cannabis medicine should not be used in children unless potential benefits outweigh theoretical risks. This same standard should apply to any medication used by children.

Cannabis Use Disorder

Another potential concern with cannabis use is that it could lead to either substance abuse or a cannabis use disorder linked with apathetic or amotivational behaviour. A substance use disorder is a persistent and recurrent use of a substance despite adverse effects on normal life and function. Part of the challenge in assessing the data in these areas is that many or most people with cannabis use issues also choose to use other drugs, including alcohol. This mixing of inebriants makes it difficult to define the specific role of cannabis in these disorders, but current estimates are that regular recreational cannabis users have approximately a 9 percent chance of developing a substance abuse problem as defined in the Diagnostic and Statistical Manual of Mental Disorders, 5th Edition (DSM-5).[54] This likelihood would give recreational cannabis a lower risk of substance abuse potential than alcohol, benzodiazepines, and opioids but still enough to be taken seriously. We currently don't have data on any abuse potential of the lower-THC or non-THC medical cannabis medicines.

Other Chronic Side Effects

Long-term recreational cannabis use in adolescents has also been linked to lower academic test scores, lower IQ, slightly lower cognitive function, and increased risk of depression and suicide. However, the data become less clear when confounding variables are considered. Closer evaluation of the evidence suggests that individuals who choose to be frequent cannabis users may have genetic, behavioural, and other environmental risk factors that might cause lower functioning and future adverse outcomes even if they didn't use cannabis. However, recent data does show that cannabis abstinence in previous teenage cannabis users results in improved verbal learning scores, suggesting cannabis use in youth likely does interfere with cognitive function to some degree. A study published in early 2019 associated adolescent recreational cannabis consumption with increased risk of developing depression and suicidal behavior later in life.[55] While not considered proof of a causal link due to possible confounding variables, this study gives increasing support to the notion that recreational cannabis use in youth should be strongly discouraged.

CONTRAINDICATIONS

In medicine, a contraindication is a reason that a drug should not be used. There are very few absolute contraindications for any medical cannabis product. Despite extensive use by people with nearly every medical condition, there have been no verified cannabis deaths. I am always amazed when colleagues say they won't endorse cannabis because of possible risks. We accept significant risks in modern medicine with most current pharmaceuticals. Cannabis, like all other medicines, does have risks. It just so happens that cannabis has far fewer risks than most. Still, in some situations, cannabis is not suitable, and patients with one of the relative contraindications to cannabis should not receive cannabis authorization from a health care provider in Canada unless benefits of therapy clearly outweigh risks. Also worth noting is that currently all contraindications are listed for cannabis medicine as a whole, with no separate contraindications for THC, CBD, or other specific cannabinoids. Although we know different cannabinoids produce different effects, and therefore pose different risks, they are all grouped together for the purpose of these recommendations and will continue to be until we collect more specific safety data.

The College of Family Physicians of Canada outlines the following conditions for which cannabis is not appropriate unless potential benefits outweigh potential risks: the person is (1) under twenty-five years of age, (2) has a personal or family history of psychosis, (3) has a current or past cannabis use disorder or active substance abuse disorder, (4) has significant cardiovascular or respiratory disease.[56] Health Canada publishes a similar but more extensive list, recommending cannabis not be used unless benefits clearly outweigh risks in the following situations: (1) patients who are under eighteen years of age, (2) patients who are allergic to cannabis, (3) patients with serious liver, kidney, heart, or lung disease, (4) patients with a personal or family history of psychotic mental conditions, such as schizophrenia, (5) patients with a personal history of substance abuse, (6) women who are pregnant or breastfeeding, and (7) men wishing to start a family.[57] Let's take a closer look at these scenarios.

Children and Teens

In pediatric medicine, safety is always considered to be of paramount importance. Even small potential risks have to be considered when patients have long projected lives ahead of them. Therefore, even though we lack safety data on use of specific medical cannabis products in children, the emphasis is on caution and safety. There is a general consensus that the effects of cannabis on the actively growing brain are poorly understood and that brain development can continue up to the age of twenty-five. Additionally, a number of studies have associated use of recreational cannabis by youth as a risk factor for poor school performance and general amotivational behaviour. Therefore, most guidelines advocate avoiding cannabis use in individuals under twenty-five and particularly in those under age eighteen, though guidelines vary among organizations and between provincial and federal governments.

Governmental recommendations across Canada vary by province and territory, though most reference Health Canada's guidelines. Those guidelines state a minimum appropriate age of eighteen, specifying that benefits may outweigh risks in a small number of cases. Due to concerns about potential effects of cannabis on the developing brain, the College of Physicians and Surgeons of Ontario is more conservative than Health Canada and is clear about the potential harm of prescribing to patients under twenty-five. As for the other provinces, British Columbia's guidelines state that cannabis is generally not appropriate for patients under age eighteen but that medical decisions should be made after analysis of risks versus benefits. The Alberta College references the age eighteen limit as described in the Health Canada document and also emphasizes the importance of an evaluation of risks versus benefits. The Saskatchewan guidelines do not specifically refer to age limits but do reference the Health Canada document. In Manitoba, the guidelines state that a health care provider should make a conventional diagnosis using the principles of good medical care, but an age limit is not specifically discussed. In Quebec, guidelines suggest avoiding use under twenty-five years of age, except in special medical circumstances. Other provinces and territories lack specific local age recommendations. They either reference the Health Canada document, or formal cannabis policy is still being revised.

The recent recreational legalization poses another consideration for prescribing medical cannabis to younger patients. Since most Canadian provinces have set the legal age limit for recreational cannabis to eighteen or nineteen, defending an age limit of twenty-five for cannabis medicine may be difficult. This higher age limit for medical cannabis is particularly problematic since potential harms of cannabis mostly apply to high-THC recreational products, which could be more easily accessed than safer medicinal products for young Canadians. However, it's important to remember that while recreational age limits are actual legal limits, the medical age "limits" are simply recommendations. Health care providers are legally allowed to authorize medical cannabis to a patient of any age as long as they can justify that their medical decision-making process has evaluated risks versus benefits.

Therefore, despite numerous guidelines, even for pediatric patients the potential benefits of medical cannabis sometimes outweigh risks. For parents with children suffering from severe intractable epilepsy, for example, or other diseases unresponsive to conventional therapy, the advice to not use cannabis in patients under twenty-five years of age may seem ridiculous. In fact, drug-resistant pediatric epilepsy has shown significant response to cannabis treatments. Since the 2017 study reporting favourable results was published in the *New England Journal of Medicine*,[41] parents of children with drug-resistant epilepsy have stepped forward and requested that legal cannabis treatment be available. It was, in fact, many of these same families, who had previously reported remarkable improvements in their epileptic children with use of unregulated high-CBD cannabis prior to legalization, who spurred some of the official research and legalization efforts.

Consequently, most specialist neurologist physicians will recommend cannabis medicine for children if benefits are deemed to outweigh risks. Most health care providers would also agree that a twenty-year-old patient with drug-resistant chemotherapy-induced nausea and vomiting or severe opioid-resistant pain from any cause should at least have the benefit of an evaluation and an opinion. The decision to use medical cannabis must ultimately be made between an experienced health care provider and the patient and family.

In summary, I will stress that there is no prohibition against a health care provider making an educated risk-benefit analysis for use of cannabis medicine in a patient of any age. As in any other area of medicine, every patient should be evaluated on the basis of medical need and a patient-specific risk-benefit evaluation. A refusal to evaluate any patient under age eighteen is not good medicine. Each patient situation should be evaluated separately. Just as some older patients don't meet criteria for medical cannabis, some patients eighteen and younger do. The existing guidelines stress that patients should be evaluated and therapy recommended if benefits outweigh risks.

Pregnancy

Cannabis has not been proven safe for pregnant women, and those who are pregnant, trying to get pregnant, or breastfeeding are strongly advised to avoid all cannabis products to ensure the sound development of the fetus and infant. We don't know of any specific harms to the fetus from cannabis exposure, other than possible low birth weight, though animal studies have suggested possible adverse effect on brain development. These two potential harms alone are enough reason to recommend against cannabis use in pregnancy, and we don't have enough data to support use in pregnancy or breastfeeding either. Therefore, to stay on the side of safety, cannabis use should be avoided in pregnant women or in women who are trying to get pregnant.

The Canadian and US obstetrics and gynecology societies both provide official recommendations. The official statement of the Society of Obstetricians and Gynecologists of Canada is as follows:

> Cannabis (marijuana) is the most commonly used illicit drug among pregnant women. Legalization of cannabis in Canada may reinforce the reputation of cannabis being a harmless drug and result in an increase of use among pregnant women.
>
> Evidence-based data has shown that cannabis use during pregnancy can adversely affect the growth and development of the baby, and may lead to long-term learning and behavioural consequences. There have been sufficient studies with comparable results, showing that cannabis use during pregnancy raises concerns of impaired neurodevelopment of the fetus, in addition to the adverse health consequences related to maternal and fetal exposure to the effects of smok-

ing. Pregnancy is a critical time for the brain development of the baby and the adverse effects caused by cannabis exposure can be life-long.

The [Society of Obstetricians and Gynecologists of Canada] recommends that women who are pregnant or contemplating pregnancy should abstain from cannabis use during pregnancy.[58]

The American College of Obstetricians and Gynecologists provides similar guidance:

Before pregnancy and in early pregnancy, all women should be asked about their use of tobacco, alcohol, and other drugs, including marijuana and other medications used for non-medical reasons. Women reporting marijuana use should be counseled about concerns regarding potential adverse health consequences of continued use during pregnancy.

Women who are pregnant or contemplating pregnancy should be encouraged to discontinue marijuana use. Pregnant women or women contemplating pregnancy should be encouraged to discontinue use of marijuana for medicinal purposes in favor of an alternative therapy for which there are better pregnancy-specific safety data. There are insufficient data to evaluate the effects of marijuana use on infants during lactation and breastfeeding, and in the absence of such data, cannabis use is discouraged.[59]

Therefore, in both Canada and the United States, the official guidelines are clear. Do not use cannabis if you are pregnant or trying to become pregnant. While there is no strong evidence that cannabis is particularly dangerous in these situations, there is also no evidence that it's safe, and it may cause harm.

Despite the fact that it's not recommended, many women do admit to using cannabis while pregnant. In one California study, almost 10 percent of pregnant women admitted to using cannabis.[60] Use was usually episodic to relieve morning sickness, but some women used cannabis to relax since any alcohol use in pregnancy is considered unacceptable. In some US states, severe pregnancy-related nausea and vomiting is considered an appropriate indication for cannabis if authorized by a health care provider. In Canada, the recommendation is that it should not be used unless strong potential benefits outweigh risks.

Establishing the true risk of a medication in pregnancy is very difficult. It's unethical to randomize pregnant women to exposure of a drug in order to determine what might happen to the developing fetus. Therefore, most of the evidence with regard to cannabis use in pregnancy comes from observational studies of women who admit to using cannabis during pregnancy and comparing their fetal outcomes against women who said they did not use cannabis. Unfortunately, these studies are difficult to interpret since it's often difficult to rule out the effects of other factors, such as whether alcohol or other drugs were used, whether the patient had other illness that affected the pregnancy, and the type, strength, and dose of cannabis taken. We also know that a lot of street cannabis is contaminated, and contaminants may also contribute to harms. Ultimately, there is no conclusive proof that smoking or consuming cannabis will or will not significantly harm a growing fetus. We also have no data on risks of medical cannabis products, which may have very different effects than typical recreational products, in pregnancy. Therefore, because we don't know for sure, it's important to make recommendations on the assumption that cannabis may harm the fetus and send a message that no cannabis use in pregnancy is recommended.

Fertility

Data is conflicting with regard to the effect of cannabis use on fertility. We don't have any data on medical cannabis products specifically, but evidence suggests that regular use of recreational cannabis can lower sperm count and decrease testosterone in men. On the other hand, evidence suggests that cannabis may enhance libido and sexual desire, particularly in women, so the overall data on conception and fertility is mixed. Also, because we have evidence that regular recreational cannabis use in pregnant women can cause low-birthweight infants, it's not supposed to be used while trying to get pregnant. Therefore, even though we don't know the true effect of cannabis on fertility, the recommendation from most fertility experts is that couples who are trying to conceive should stop using it.

Renal, Hepatic, Cardiac, Lung Disease

One of the contraindications to cannabis listed by Health Canada is the presence of serious renal, hepatic, cardiac, or lung disease. Defining the word *serious* is problematic as there will be inevitable subjectivity and grey areas. Typically in medicine, a serious disease is one that could produce significant limitations to normal function or life expectancy. The take-home message should be that in any patient with significant disease of any vital organ system, great care should be taken when adding any new therapy or medication that could potentially worsen the pre-existing disease. As with many areas of cannabis medicine, we are lacking comprehensive evidence to guide therapy, but overall a harm-reduction and avoidance approach should be emphasized.

In terms of kidney disease, we know that CB1 and CB2 receptors are present in renal tissue, so we can theorize that cannabis would have an effect on the kidney. Currently, however, we lack data to show whether these effects are beneficial or deleterious in the presence of pre-existing kidney disease. Most existing studies have shown no appreciable effects of cannabis on normal kidney function, but in the situation of renal failure or renal transplantation, we don't know what effects might be.[61] Cannabis use should therefore be considered only if benefits outweigh risks and after consultation with a nephrologist.

Essentially the same situation exists when discussing the use of cannabis medicine in patients with severe existing liver disease. Ultimately, we do not know for sure. We know that CB1 and CB2 receptors are present in the liver, but their exact roles in health and disease are poorly understood. Evidence appears to be accumulating that cannabis may actually be beneficial in patients with some forms of hepatic disease. More than one recent study has shown that cannabis use is associated with a lower risk of liver disease in alcoholics and may help stimulate repair mechanisms in damaged hepatic cells.[62,63] Given these possible benefits, we may be close to actually recommending cannabis to patients with some forms of liver disease. In the meantime, the recommendation remains that cannabis should be used in the presence of severe hepatic disease only if benefits outweigh risks and after consultation with an experienced hepatologist.

Recreational cannabis is known to produce variable changes to blood pressure, including both temporary spikes and dips in blood pressure. Patients with severe postural hypotension or severe hypertension may therefore be at risk. No validated data has looked at the effects of specific medical cannabis preparations on blood pressure, but the advice for any patient with fragile blood pressure problems is that cannabis medicine should be used only under the care and monitoring of an experienced health care provider.

Cardiac disease remains the largest killer of North Americans and is incredibly common in the general population. Even in the absence of confirmatory data, any medicine that might potentially worsen existing cardiac disease should be avoided. Therefore, the standard recommendation is that cannabis should not be used by patients with severe heart disease. However, once again there is conflicting and inconclusive evidence regarding the role of cannabis in cardiac disease and almost no data on effects of non-inhaled medical cannabis. We know that cannabis can transiently increase heart rate, and yet evidence that cannabis contributes adversely to rate-dependent coronary perfusion is limited. Of multiple studies on the cardiovascular effects of cannabis, some showed risk, some showed benefit, and some showed no appreciable positive or negative effect. Until we have more conclusive data, the recommendation is to avoid cannabis use in patients with severe cardiac disease unless benefits outweigh risks and use only after consultation with a cardiologist.

Patients with severe lung disease are usually in a fragile physical state that may be easily disrupted. Therefore, any new medication, including cannabis, must be used with caution. Much of the concern related to cannabis use in patients with lung disease relates to the harms of smoking and the risk of exacerbating existing airspace disease. It seems like a fairly obvious recommendation to say that patients with severe lung disease should not smoke cannabis, or any-thing else for that matter. Not surprisingly, both the Lung Association of Canada and the American Thoracic Society recommend that people with lung disease do not smoke cannabis.[64,65] There has, however, never been conclusive evidence that smoking cannabis contributes to lung cancer. Interestingly, certain strains of cannabis are reported by patients to improve their chronic obstructive pulmonary disease (COPD) symptoms and make breathing easier. We know that com-ponents of cannabis are anti-inflammatory and airway dilators, so the reported improvements are certainly plausible. Cannabis inhalers and nebulizers could therefore likely become treatments for lung dis-ease in the future. However, smoking is not recommended for medical cannabis use, as there are safer and more precise mechanisms for inhalational therapy. Use of cannabis in patients with severe lung disease should only be considered with input from an experienced pulmonary specialist.

Regardless of which vital organ system we're talking about, pa-tients with severe organ disease are likely to be taking multiple other medicines. Some of these medications have very narrow effective ranges and can clash with other medicines. In the next section, I dis-cuss potential medication interactions with cannabis in more detail. The take-home message is that while no known drugs are absolutely contraindicated with cannabis, any medication taken for manage-ment of severe, life-threatening disease must be used cautiously with cannabis and only under the supervision of an experienced physician.

Interactions with Other Medications

All medicines have potential interactions. Sometimes these are trivial and harmless, and other times they are serious and dangerous. As with any medical therapy, it's important to think about the possible ways cannabis may interact with other medications. Therefore, it's also important for patients to disclose all current medications to their health care provider, including use of medical cannabis. Currently, we have almost no data evaluating how specific medical cannabis preparations interact with existing pharmaceuticals, but we do have some data regarding effects of recreational cannabis.

The nature of interactions depends on the type and quantity of both the medication and the cannabis. In some cases, cannabis may increase or decrease the effectiveness or potency of other drugs. Cannabis products may also interfere with how other drugs are metabolized due to interaction with their metabolism in the liver. Caution is therefore required when using any medication that has delicate hepatic metabolism. Even if the interaction of cannabis and other medication is potentially beneficial, close monitoring by a medical professional along with regular blood work, when indicated, is important. While a common worry might be that cannabis may cause other medicines to stop working, in some cases, cannabis may actually increase the effectiveness or potency of other drugs. This potentiating effect could be either positive or negative, depending on the situation. For many drugs, increased potency would be undesirable as it usually also means increased side effects. This situation is particularly true for blood pressure medications, blood thinners, opioid narcotics, insulin, and any potent sedatives.

Blood Thinners

While reports of adverse events related to cannabis and blood thinner medications (anticoagulation medications, such as warfarin and heparin) are rare, cannabis has been known to compound the effects of these medications in some situations. For patients on blood thinners, significant caution is advised. The effect of cannabis on these medications has been reported to be variable and is not well studied. Usually, close monitoring is required and a risk-benefit discussion should be had prior to initiating cannabis therapy. In reality, many medical cannabis patients are on anticoagulation medication, and adverse outcomes are rare. However, due to the serious potential consequences of either over or under anticoagulation, a cautious approach is indicated.

Insulin

As with many areas of cannabis medicine, evidence on the effects of cannabis on diabetic patients is mixed, and interactions with oral hypoglycemics and insulin are not well defined. Mounting evidence suggests that cannabis use may cause less insulin resistance and improved insulin response, particularly in pre-diabetes and type 2 diabetes.[66] While type 1 diabetic cannabis users typically report no change in insulin use or blood sugars, caution is advised and careful blood sugar monitoring is indicated when starting new medication.

Opioids

When combined with opioid or sedative medications, cannabis may produce an additive effect causing marked sedation. This effect appears to be particularly true for high-THC products, but we lack data for the low-THC/high-CBD medicines. Patients already taking drugs with a strong potential sedative effect, including alcohol, opioids, benzodiazepines, barbiturates, and narcotics, should avoid cannabis unless directed by a health care provider. The medications propoxyphene and buprenorphine have been specifically linked to a risk of over sedation when used with cannabis, and patients are advised to avoid cannabis when taking these medications.

CHAPTER 6
EVIDENCE OF EFFECTIVENESS

In this chapter, I'll attempt to summarize the existing evidence that either supports or refutes the benefits of medical cannabis. One of the reasons many Canadian physicians still don't feel comfortable authorizing medical cannabis is that they weren't taught about it in medical school, and they weren't introduced to it in the traditional manner used to introduce new drugs. Typically, when a new drug is brought to market, physicians learn about it when findings of a new major drug trial are published. Pharmaceutical representatives then spend months or years visiting hospitals and offices presenting stacks of papers and scientific evidence supporting the new drug. That's not how modern cannabis medicine was introduced. Cannabis medicine came back in Canada as a result of patients demanding access and winning cases in court, and pharmaceutical companies have not been at the helm of its resurgence. Consequently, physicians were not given the opportunity to learn about cannabis in a conventional way.

THE TROUBLE WITH (INTERPRETING) CANNABIS RESEARCH

The practice of medicine is already so complicated and difficult that most doctors depend on the established process outlined above for introducing new drugs. When this process didn't happen with cannabis, doctors started to push back by stating that there is no evidence that medical cannabis works. While this statement is simply not true, it's understandable that many doctors are uncomfortable trying to wade through the large quantity of variable-quality cannabis data that we do have. Due to this reality, doctors depend on their professional societies to interpret data for them. Unfortunately, the professional societies are also struggling to interpret the existing cannabis research.

An example of the challenge facing doctors and their societies was highlighted in February 2018 when the College of Family Physicians of Canada attempted to summarize the existing medical cannabis data. The review article, "Systematic Review of Systematic Reviews for Medical Cannabinoids," examined evidence for medical cannabis use in three areas for which most cannabis research had been previously performed: pain, spasticity, and nausea and vomiting.[67] The paper concluded that the most common effects of cannabis were negative side effects and that there was little conclusive evidence to support widespread medical cannabis use. These conclusions were confusing to many doctors and patients. If there is established current and historical evidence of successful medical cannabis use, why would the journal of the College of Family Physicians of Canada reach these conclusions?

The truth is, medical cannabis is not supported by conventional large-scale research data, which is the way most new pharmaceutical drugs are evaluated. The published review by the college only looked for these large conventional studies, a typical approach to systematic meta-analysis. Finding none, the authors concluded that there was insufficient evidence. However, more than twenty thousand published papers that examine cannabis are listed on PubMed, a searchable journal database. Yet the majority of these published studies do not meet criteria for inclusion into a systematic review of large trials, such as the recent college review. Ultimately, only thirty-one papers met criteria for consideration. Unfortunately, no rigorous large, phased, step-wise drug trials were available for cannabis, and therefore the paper concluded that there was a lack of evidence of benefit.

The lack of large conventional drug trials in cannabis medicine exists for a number of reasons, some of which I've already mentioned. A lot of the challenge has to do with money, and large US-based corporations drive much of the world's pharmaceutical research. No single company has been in a position to profit from patented cannabis sales, and, therefore, no company has invested the hundreds of millions of dollars such trials require. Additionally, a century of prohibition has made rigorous cannabis research almost impossible. Schedule I status in the United States essentially guarantees no large-scale quality research can occur there as research on prohibited substances is strictly curtailed. Trying to do cannabis research under the Schedule I status requires literally years of applications and paperwork and, if finally approved, using only a single government-controlled source of cannabis for research. That cannabis is of dubious consistency and quality, making results questionable anyway.

TYPES OF EVIDENCE

In order to understand the current state of cannabis research and how health care providers make informed decisions about which medicines to prescribe, it will be helpful to first take a look at the conventional process for evaluating medicines and the types of evidence that providers look for. Standard pharmaceuticals typically go through a predictable and rigorous set of evaluations that include preclinical and clinical trials. These large studies are referred to as phased, step-wise drug trials and are usually performed before a medicine is brought to market.

Phases of Clinical Trials

Drug studies usually begin in the laboratory with proof of potential efficacy in cell cultures and animal models. These studies are called preclinical since they do not involve investigation of clinical effects on humans. This stage of investigation typically lasts three to five years. If these preclinical studies provide proof of likely efficacy and safety, an application for human studies is required. If approved, the drug enters into what is known as a phase I study, which examines the effects of the medicine on healthy human volunteers. During this phase, the safety and basic effects of the drug, like absorption, metabolism, and excretion, are studied. Typically between fifty and one hundred volunteers are required, and these studies take one to two years.

If phase I studies demonstrate acceptable safety, then phase II studies are conducted, where patients with the disease in question volunteer to take the experimental medication and researchers try to determine the effectiveness of the drug at varying doses or concentrations. Phase II studies typically involve hundreds of volunteers and take two to three years. If a drug has demonstrated safety and efficacy in phases I and II, it can enter a phase III study, which is a large, randomized trial run over many years in order to examine whether the new drug works better than the best treatment already available, or a placebo if no treatment is available for comparison. These phase III trials usually involve thosuands of patients and are performed at many hopsitals and clinics in order to recruit enough patients for the study (known as a multi-centre study design). Phase III trials usually take many years to complete and are typically incredibly expensive to run from start to finish. They're usually funded by large pharmaceutical companies that are hoping to patent an effective and profitable medicine.

After completion of a successful phase III trial, drugs can be brought to market but are then subject to years of post-marketing surveillance that looks at long-term efficacy, cost effectiveness, delayed side effects, and other factors. It usually takes twelve to fifteen years to take a drug from preclinical studies into this phase IV surveillance. While the above-outlined process is typical for new drugs, cannabis existed as a medicine and was being used by humans thousands of years before the development of modern drug trials. It wasn't discovered as a potential new drug by modern research scientists and subsequently was never examined by phased drug trials. It's important to undertand that formal drug trials are only one component of medical research. Not all clinical research involves introduction of a newly discovered drug, and most therapeutic studies occur outside of the rigid phased drug trial format.

Types of Studies

The gold-standard for high-quality therapeutic research is the randomized controlled trial (RCT), and as mentioned these are included in phase III of standard drug trials. RCTs are referred to as *randomized* since the patient groups studied are randomly selected from among all participants. Each participant is randomly assigned to receive either the study drug, a conventional standard treatment, or a placebo (inactive drug). The word *control* refers to the fact that the study drug is compared to a placebo or conventional treatment control.

Of course, researchers perform other less-rigourous trials that also provide valuable evidence. In fact, the majority of evidence in medicine comes from these lower-level studies since they are easier and less costly to perform, and they enable scientists to examine rare events for which not enough patients could be gathered for a randomized study. These studies include cohort studies, case-control studies, case series, and cross-sectional studies. A cohort study follows a group of patients with a specific risk factor or trait over time and compares its outcome to a control group that does not have the risk factor. A case-control study compares a group of patients with a specific outcome to a matched set of patients without the outcome and looks backward in time, or retrospectively, to determine possible risk factors or events that may have caused the disease. A case series is a detailed report and analysis on a group of patients with a certain disease without comparing to a control group, and a cross-sectional study is a comprehensive review of data pertaining to a population at a specific point in time. I encourage interested readers to continue exploring these subjects online or through groups, such as the Centre for Evidence-Based Medicine at the University of Oxford.[68]

Levels of Evidence

The very best available scientific evidence is considered to be a conclusive, systematic, statistical analysis of multiple statistically significant RCTs, particularly if the analyzed trials have homogeneous or similar results. In plain language, this means that if multiple large, well-conducted studies all have the same result, then the results are likely to be true. In the medical science community, this breadth of support is considered level 1a evidence, and we currently have no level 1a evidence in cannabis medicine. Large trials that would significantly contribute to level 1a evidence are prohibitively expensive, often costing hundreds of millions of dollars, and are almost always funded by industry that intends to patent a profitable new product. In cannabis medicine, they may never occur.

The next level of scientific evidence, good but not ideal, is considered level 1b. Less powerful level 1b evidence would be a single RCT with statistically significant results and narrow confidence intervals, meaning a high level of accuracy. There is currently some, but minimal, level 1b evidence in cannabis medicine. It's the relative lack of this higher-level 1a and 1b evidence that leads some physicians and professional groups to say, "There is not enough evidence in cannabis medicine."

Most evidence in cannabis medicine is currently from expert opinion, case series, cohort trials, or smaller, low-quality RCTs. These types of data are considered levels 2, 3, and 4 evidence. It turns out that much of modern conventional medical practice is supported by only levels 2, 3, and 4 evidence. The fact that we don't have level 1 evidence for a medical therapy or drug does not prove lack of efficacy. It means only that more prospective RCTs are required before the medical community is willing to say, "There is enough evidence."

This lack of higher-level conclusive evidence may seem discouraging from the outset, but an overwhelming amount of the evidence we do have, including thousands of studies and thousands of years of use, points to the safety and efficacy of cannabis in a wide (indeed, surprisingly so) range of clinical settings. The existing evidence highlights a spectacular safety profile and minimal unwanted side effects. Really, with cannabis, we already have the most important data, which is long-term clinical data showing safety and efficacy. These types of data normally come *after* initial drug trials. We have five thousand years of real-world data for cannabis, which is incredibly valuable, but we do not have the conventional phased drug trials that normally occur before introduction of a new pharmaceutical.

These phased drug trials usually precede the phase IV long-term safety and efficacy data. Instead, in many ways, we have the data gathering backward with cannabis. We have the phase IV long-term safety and efficacy data, but we don't have the phase I, II, and III preceding trials. Whether we go backward and complete these specific trials for cannabis is a matter of debate. I suspect it's unrealistic and not financially feasible. Ultimately, however, a sufficient amount of research will likely emerge from the evolving legal, social, and financial reforms accompanying cannabis legalization.

CURRENT STATE OF CANNABIS RESEARCH

Due to the cost and difficulty of rigourous medical research, it will likely take many years before significant new medical cannabis data emerges. In the meantime, while there is concensus that more prospective high-quality RCTs are required in cannabis medicine, in order to make an evidenced-based decision, a health care provider must consider the preponderance of evidence that currently exists.

As a former practicing surgeon, I had to acknowledge that a large amount of surgery I performed was not supported by rigorous medical data. In fact, by some estimates, less than 30 percent of surgical work is supported by conclusive scientific evidence. The rest is accumulated surgical wisdom and data from observational or non-randomized research. If physicians had to hold surgery up to evaluation by meta-analysis of large RCTs, they would not be able to practise as surgeons.

The same decision-making process applies to most areas of medicine. Day-to-day medical practice is often based on wisdom and habit accumulated by previous generations of providers rather than simply on the results of RCTs. Most medical practice would not stand up to rigorous statistical analysis. The same is true for many medications we use. If opioid medications, for example, were currently held up to such standards, their use would be abolished.

In medicine, we should look at the totality of the facts and circumstances. For cannabis, our understanding includes more than five thousand years of documented effective human use, more than twenty thousand published studies, including many smaller RCTs, and an incredible safety profile. As already stated many times, there has never been a verified death from cannabis. The "significant" cannabis harms mentioned in the 2018 Family Practice review article were almost entirely the results of temporary intoxication with THC and included dizziness, impaired coordination, and altered mood. Not surprisingly, since most published studies predate the newer, non-psychoactive medical cannabinoids, patients were "high." The studies did not document any deaths or truly serious, life-threatening adverse events. It's hard to understand how temporary inebriation is a "significant" harm.

As mentioned, it's challenging for Canadian family physicians to endorse cannabis when their own college publishes a review stating that cannabis poses significant harms. They reached this conclusion despite the lack of any reported serious adverse outcomes. The same cannot be said of most drug trials of existing pharmaceuticals. One of the studies included in the recent meta-analysis states that "use of existing medical cannabinoids appears to increase the risk of non-serious adverse events."[44] In other words, common side effects like dizziness are common, but there is no proof that cannabis causes any serious long-term harms. Common over-the-counter medicines, like Benadryl (diphenhydramine) and Gravol (dimenhydrinate), list side effects that are very similar to the ones listed for cannabis, including dizziness and impaired coordination. It's unclear why cannabis is judged so differently.

MISINTERPRETATION OF THE DATA

Based on the fact that cannabis is at least as safe as, and likely safer than, most of our current commonly used medications, I find that some recent professional society recommendations on cannabis are gross misinterpretations of the available data. As an example, I found the College of Family Physicians recommendation that cannabis not be used as a first- or second-line agent in palliative care shocking. Palliative patients have incurable disease and are often suffering. They are frequently given strong medicines with significant side effects in order to control their symptoms. Why should use of cannabis be different? Would any health care provider tell a dying patient they shouldn't have a glass of wine because they might get dizzy or drunk? Of course not, yet alcohol causes thousands of deaths and huge morbidity across North America every year. Would any provider tell palliative patients that they shouldn't take pain medicine because they might get drowsy? Of course not, yet the prescription opioid crisis takes tens of thousands of lives per year. Cannabis helps palliative patients with pain, sleep, depression, and anxiety. Patients can decide how much and how often they use cannabis, giving them control over how they choose to live and medicate. Suggesting they not use it due to the possibility of minor temporary side effects is both unethical and absurd.

While evidence does support medical cannabis efficacy, interpreting it unfortunately takes extra work for health care providers. It's much easier to rely on the guidance of individual professional colleges. Thankfully, for both patients and their providers, a separate review of the benefits of cannabis in palliative care was published in June 2018 in the *Annals of Palliative Medicine*.[69] This paper concluded that cannabis-based medicines were likely going to become increasingly important in the control of a wide range of bothersome symptoms in the palliative patient. This review showed the results of a survey of US oncologists where 67 percent viewed cannabis as an effective adjunct to standard pain therapies in their palliative cancer patients.[70] Results of an Israeli study were also reported where 69.5 percent of palliative patients reported good quality of life after six months of medical cannabis therapy as opposed to only 18.7 percent before cannabis therapy.[71]

Evidence supporting cannabis continues to accumulate, with recent studies demonstrating effectiveness of cannabis in treating multiple conditions, which I review in more detail in Chapter 8. Published papers include a thorough and inclusive review of medical cannabis evidence, published in 2017 by the National Academies of Sciences, Engineering, and Medicine. Its main findings were that "there is conclusive or substantial evidence that cannabis or cannabinoids are effective for the treatment of chronic pain in adults, as antiemetics in the treatment of chemotherapy-induced nausea and vomiting, and for improving patient-reported multiple sclerosis spasticity symptoms."[72] For all other health conditions, reviewers determined that current available evidence was moderate or limited. For many areas of human disease, evidence supporting the use of cannabis was inconclusive.

However, as a sign of how quickly cannabis science is progressing, while the National Academies report put epilepsy in the "inconclusive evidence" category, only two months later a pivotal paper demonstrating efficacy of cannabinoids in the treatment of pediatric epilepsy was published in the *New England Journal of Medicine*.[41] Results of this RCT showed that cannabis medicine had a statistically significant benefit in the treatment of drug-resistant pediatric seizure disorders. That paper alone had tremendous influence on health care providers and policy makers. It resulted in approval by the FDA of the first cannabinoid medicine in the United States, a CBD extract called Epidiolex, which became officially available by prescription on November 1, 2018. As we enter into this new era of more widespread cannabis acceptance and legalization, the volume of cannabis research is set to skyrocket and health care providers will have significantly more data to answer relevant clinical questions.

Ultimately, the answer to, "Does medical cannabis work?" really depends on how the question is evaluated. Today, if you ask the more than three hundred thousand patients who have already accessed legal medical cannabis in Canada, you would hear that cannabis helps them with chronic pain, sleep disorders, anxiety, PTSD, headaches, and menstrual cramps, among many more conditions. They would tell you that medical cannabis works.

Under the lens of conventional statistical evaluation of large RCTs or meta-analysis of systematic reviews, however, you might get a different answer. The existing evidence supporting cannabis medicine primarily shows benefit in chronic pain, chemotherapy-induced nausea and vomiting, pain and spasticity of multiple sclerosis, and drug-resistant pediatric epilepsy. Even among these conditions there is still debate. An October 2018 systematic review in the journal *Pain* concluded that the current evidence doesn't clearly support cannabis use for non-cancer pain.[73] The truth is that rigorous medical data for most conditions is lacking when evaluated from this perspective. However, dozens of additional trials are currently underway, including a conventional phase III trial of cannabis in the treatment of PTSD. In the next five years, we should have significant additional supportive data of cannabis efficacy in multiple human conditions. There is also a major push to develop more non-psychoactive cannabis medicines, which should mitigate some of the common THC-related side effects.

FUTURE OF CANNABIS RESEARCH

As for why we lack more rigorous medical cannabis studies, I've already reviewed the financial, legal, and cultural factors that have been inhibiting research efforts for decades. In addition to these reasons, it also may not have occurred to researchers to investigate the effects of cannabis on such a diverse range of conditions until the evidence for the ECS and cannabinoid receptors throughout the body had been discovered and disseminated. With increased understanding of the biochemical composition of the plant and discovery of how these compounds work within our body, more avenues of research are now open to investigate the implications of these findings.

The future of cannabis research is now, and it's an exciting time for medical cannabis science. Rigorous research depends on two primary factors: adequate monetary funding and a favourable academic and regulatory environment. For the first time ever, these two factors are converging. The Canadian government recently announced millions of dollars of funding, and academic institutions are scrambling to submit grant applications. Canadian LPs have seen public enthusiasm for cannabis and cannabis stocks skyrocket, resulting in a massive infusion of capital that's starting to be invested in research and development. Further afield, the University of Oxford boasts a new medical cannabis research program, and academic cannabis research is underway at multiple University of California campuses, including UC Davis and a multidisciplinary cannabis institute, the UCI Center for the Study of Cannabis, at UC Irvine.

Overall, this influx of money and interest will likely cause an explosion of research into the effects of multiple cannabis compounds on human disease. Recently planned trials, and some currently active ones, will examine the effects of cannabis on chronic pain, anxiety, fibromyalgia, essential tremor, autoimmune disease, osteoarthritis, PTSD, autism spectrum disorder, and insomnia. Ongoing trials in Israel are looking at the effects of various cannabinoid preparations on human cancer cell lines. Furthermore, jurisdictions around the world where cannabis has been legalized in some capacity are beginning to yield enormous amounts of anecdotal and prospective clinical data, spurring an effort to observe and document both positive and negative results. In Canada particularly, this research will continue and accelerate for both medical and recreational products now that federal legalization has occurred.

PART III
TREATING WITH MEDICAL CANNABIS

We've already discussed how cannabis medicine shows promise for relief of many diseases and symptoms. However, we continue to hear from skeptics that there is no evidence that medical cannabis works. And, as discussed in Part II, the answer to the question, "Does medical cannabis work?" depends on how we interpret the current evidence. Medical cannabis is not supported by enough large-scale research data to withstand statistical scrutiny except for a few specific conditions. Even in those conditions, the level 1a evidence (systematic reviews of large trials with consistent results) is still lacking. The areas for which we have the best evidence of cannabis efficacy are chronic pain, chemotherapy-induced nausea and vomiting, pain and spasticity of multiple sclerosis, and anorexia and cachexia of HIV/AIDS. Most observers would also add relief of drug-resistant epilepsy in pediatric patients and relief of pain and suffering in palliative and oncology patients. Even though that group of diseases and symptoms for which cannabis has proven efficacy is already large and remarkably diverse, patients continue to report benefit in a wider range of symptoms. In this part of the book, I first consider some factors necessary for understanding and interpreting cannabis research. Next, I review the existing knowledge on treating thirty-eight conditions with cannabis medicine. Finally, I provide some guidelines around obtaining, authorizing, and dosing medical cannabis.

CHAPTER 7

CONSIDERATIONS FOR TREATMENT

Before starting medical cannabis treatment, it's important to acknowledge that the current approach is somewhere between conventional and natural medicines. Cannabis needs to be regulated to ensure access to clean, non-contaminated medicine of known composition. This standard is the same that applies to conventional pharmaceuticals. However, as I discuss in Chapter 9, the dosing and frequency guidelines that exist for cannabis are currently much more open and patient driven than those for most standard medicines. This situation is closer to using a natural plant supplement from a health food store. In conventional medicine, we typically use one molecular form of a drug to treat a very limited range of medical problems. In cannabis medicine, we use multiple plant compounds to treat multiple symptoms and diseases. Another unique fact about cannabis medicine is that we now have legal access in Canada to products for both recreational and medical use that come from the same plant source. Not all patients and health care providers will be comfortable with these realities, but if we keep patient safety, comfort, and quality of life as the factors of paramount importance, reaching a reasonable middle ground is possible. The following sections outline an approach to cannabis medicine that takes these realities into account and helps navigate this new ground between natural and conventional medicine.

INTERPRETING RESEARCH

If you decide to read the source material referenced in the next chapter of this book, it will be important to keep a few facts in mind as you review the current cannabis literature. First, some studies done on the effects of cannabis medicine did not use whole plant cannabis itself. Rather, they examined the effects of manufactured pharmaceutical cannabinoids and/or pharmaceutical cannabis extracts. Examples of these products are dronabinol and nabilone, synthetic forms of THC sold under the brand names Marinol and Cesamet; nabiximols, a THC and CBD extract sold under the brand name Sativex; and the recently FDA-approved CBD extract marketed as Epidiolex.

Exactly how we can apply trial results of manufactured cannabinoids to patients using whole plant cannabis medicine is not currently clear. As discussed in Chapter 4, there is suspicion, but not proof, that the entire combination of cannabis chemicals in the plant may produce a more powerful synergistic effect than individual cannabinoids alone. Therefore, trial results examining the effects of synthetic THC alone may or may not apply to treatments using whole plant product. Concentrated THC–CBD extracts may behave differently than whole plant products containing more terpenes, flavonoids, and cannabinoids. We know that pure pharmaceutical cannabinoids like nabilone do not behave exactly as whole plant ingestible oils or dry flower available from LPs behave. Even between LPs, similar whole plant products may have slightly different effects as each cannabis varietal will produce different ratios of plant chemicals. Even identical varietals won't produce the same chemical mixtures when grown under different conditions. These variables are some of the many that currently make placing cannabis medicine into the conventional pharmaceutical world difficult. Ultimately, new research efforts will need to address these many challenges.

Second, additional difficulty with the existing cannabis literature comes from the fact that the majority of published trials have evaluated smoked recreational cannabis, the source, potency, and composition of which was often unknown. How accurately the results of these trials can be applied to users of newer medical products is unclear. Finally, many previous trials recruited long-term recreational users of cannabis who may have had very different physiological responses than cannabis-naive patients. Therefore, interpreting the applicability of currently available cannabis research is difficult and is one of the reasons that many skeptics say, "There is no evidence that cannabis works." With approximately twenty thousand published cannabis studies and thousands of real-world patient success stories, there is abundant evidence cannabis works, just not yet enough large-scale evidence to satisfy some observers.

Though examining the evidence of cannabis medicine can be frustrating, this variability and difficulty in applying research data to individual patient situations is actually true to some extent in all areas of medicine. Just as no two fingerprints are identical, the interaction between a medicine and an individual patient will always be different in every case. With cannabis medicine, the variables affecting this interaction include not only how patients chose to consume the cannabis but also their personal tolerances, individual metabolisms, and what they ate or drank that day.

Because rigorous scientific research on the effects of whole plant cannabis is made even more difficult by the large number of active chemicals involved, most current research efforts are starting to evaluate limited mixtures of cannabinoids in order to try and determine which components produce therapeutic effects for specific disease states. Despite acknowledgement that whole plant cannabis might be more beneficial than individual cannabinoids alone, most research efforts are focused on the two primary cannabinoids, THC and CBD. To the frustration of patients and providers who believe in the entourage effect and additional benefits of using whole plant medicine, it likely will be many years before conventional scientific evidence is able to either validate or refute these beliefs. Once again, this reality confirms the fact that in many ways cannabis medicine still does not fit perfectly into the conventional medical model.

As a final note on interpreting these summaries, I'll provide some guidance on navigating some of the more technical scientific vocabulary you will find throughout. Though I have already discussed much of the cannabis physiology–related terminology and the types of evidence available (such as the levels of evidence and phases of trials), you may find some unfamiliar language around the designs of the studies and trials discussed. You're now familiar with the term *RCT*, which describes the standard for a high-quality clinical research trial, from Chapter 6, but you'll also want to understand some of the finer details of these RCT trials.

In addition to being randomized and controlled, most of these studies are also single, double, or fully blinded. A *single-blind* study occurs when participants don't know what drug they're receiving but researchers and analysts do. A *double-blind* study refers to a study where neither the participants nor researchers know what drug or treatment each group is being given but the analysts and statistical experts do. In a *fully-blind* study, participants, researchers, and analysts are all unaware of which treatment is being given to each group until after the study is completed and all results are calculated. In contrast, in an *open-label* study, all parties are aware of the treatments. Statistical analysis of the results of these trials is complicated, and there are organizations that specialize in this. The Cochrane group is one such organization, and it's a non-profit network of global scientists and researchers who review health care studies and data to try and guide evidence-based health care decisions. In the coming text, I mention these Cochrane reviews in several instances.

WHAT HEALTH CARE PROVIDERS NEED TO KNOW

I believe the most important thing for health care providers to know is that even though cannabis medicine is a little different from conventional medicine, it's ultimately just medicine. Cannabis is just another therapeutic tool that can help relieve symptoms in situations where potential benefits outweigh potential risks. Health care providers make these risk-benefit decisions every day. While the fact that medical cannabis can be approached with the same tools providers already use when assessing any patient may seem obvious, remembering this fact can help remove some of the apprehension that's still present among many providers.

The goal of cannabis medicine is to relieve symptoms without causing impairment and avoiding side effects, if possible. Once again, this goal is shared with all other areas of conventional medicine.

Many physicians tell me that they simply don't know enough about cannabis medicine to consider it in their practices. I often reply that they already know how to assess a patient based on a thorough history and physical. And they already know how to make a risk-benefit analysis and a patient-centred treatment decision. Therefore, prescribing cannabis medicine is subject to the same medical decision-making process used to make all treatment decisions. It involves weighing the risks and benefits of the proposed treatment in the patient being seen at that moment.

In a risk-benefit analysis, it's hard to argue that a particular treatment is risky if that treatment has never caused a verified death and has fewer side effects than most other available options. Cannabis medicine is just medicine. If physicians respond that not enough evidence supports use of cannabis in all conditions, I would reply that I agree. However, even most cannabis skeptics now acknowledge significant evidence supporting use of cannabis in chronic pain, chemotherapy-induced nausea and vomiting, pain and spasticity of multiple sclerosis, anorexia and cachexia of HIV/AIDS, drug-resistant pediatric epilepsy, and pain and suffering in both palliative and oncology patients. Hopefully agreement on this more limited list of conditions provides a common starting ground for continued academic debate around the pros and cons of medical cannabis.

I also want health care providers to know about the continuing rising demand by Canadian patients for access to safe, medically specific cannabis products. Human beings typically only pursue things that they feel are in their benefit, and people are demanding medical cannabis. This demand is not going away and will certainly grow as increasing supportive evidence evolves. Health care providers must be in a position to address this growing demand. We're moving toward refined dosing and frequency guidelines, and there's talk of placing cannabis above opioids for the treatment of chronic pain on official guidelines. Health care plans are starting to cover medical cannabis, and workplace and driving safety guidelines are being refined to address the reality of medical cannabis in the workplace and in daily life. Medical cannabis is not going away; in fact, it's growing exponentially. Initial reports are that recreational legalization has actually increased the number of Canadians seeking medically specific cannabis products. Being a Canadian health care provider at this time requires having an understanding of and an approach to cannabis medicine. It's not going away.

WHAT PATIENTS NEED TO KNOW

Patients need to know that, in Canada, they have the legal right to access safe, clean, regulated cannabis medicine to treat symptoms and diseases. They also need to know that recreational cannabis products are sold with the specific intent of producing a deliberate euphoria, relaxation, or high and that use of recreational product for medical purposes is less likely to relieve symptoms and more likely to produce impairment. The best way to use medical cannabis is with the guidance and assistance of an experienced health care provider. While finding a provider who is experienced with cannabis medicine can still be challenging, there is growing awareness and education of providers across the country. In many localities, there are also specialty medical cannabis clinics staffed by experienced physicians, nurses, and cannabis educators.

Patients also need to know which symptoms and diseases are likely to be relieved by cannabis medicine. The next chapter provides a discussion that should help. If one of the symptoms or diseases listed in Chapter 8 is your own and you are confronted with the fact that little or no evidence supports cannabis use, you should still consult with your health care provider. Your provider may decide to pursue conventional therapies until more cannabis evidence accumulates, or may decide that potential benefits of cannabis outweigh theoretical risks. The safety profile of cannabis is remarkable, and a careful trial of medical cannabis may be deemed worthwhile, particularly if you have failed to achieve symptom relief with other medications.

CHAPTER 8
SYMPTOMS AND DISEASES

In this chapter, you'll find a discussion of the effects of cannabis on some common and well-studied conditions and also on a wider range of symptoms. An exhaustive review of the literature is beyond the scope of this book, but I've attempted to provide a reasonable summary. With approximately twenty thousand published cannabis-related papers, many of them dealing with basic science questions, it's inevitable that many studies were not considered. Cannabis has potential benefit for so many symptoms and diseases that there are too many to include here, and consequently some of them were left out. Included conditions are listed in alphabetical order. After introducing each condition, I first give a brief overview of the efficacy of cannabis in treating that ailment, which will give readers a sense of our current state of knowledge. For interested readers, a summary of reviewed evidence follows along with a general outlook on future research.

All the studies mentioned are cited, with full reference information provided at the end of the book, so you can investigate the source material further if desired. One of the best summary papers on the health effects of cannabinoids was published in early 2017 by the National Academy of Sciences (hereafter referred to as the NAS review), and it's available free of charge at http://nap.edu/24625.[72] I've cited this publication multiple times and encourage interested readers to review the evidence themselves. Where appropriate, I've also tried to discuss the quality of the existing research and indicate where further research efforts are being made. However, this book is not an academic medical textbook or an exhaustively referenced treatise on cannabis medicine. I invite readers to go back to the source material or other reference publications if they want a more thorough view of the field.

These summaries should also be understood as part of an ongoing process to define and understand the medical benefits of cannabis. With so many published cannabis papers, no brief summary of cannabis research can be considered complete. New discoveries are also being made every day. In some cases, research into the effects of cannabis on a given condition may be contradictory, inconclusive, or incomplete. Those summaries may therefore be disappointing to some readers. For some symptoms or conditions, a lack of available high-quality human studies can be frustrating, with early research on mice and rats offering unclear insight into how cannabis might interact with the human body. Further research may reveal cannabis to be consistently effective as a treatment option in these cases, or it may indicate the opposite, but without rigorous research in place, scientific conclusions are impossible to reach. With these realities in mind, below you will find summaries for the diseases and conditions for which there is the most optimism for, and interest in, potential medical cannabis benefit.

ANOREXIA *see HIV/AIDS-Related Anorexia and Cachexia*

ATTENTION DISORDERS

Attention deficit disorder (ADD) and attention deficit/hyperactivity disorder (ADHD) are chronic behavioural conditions marked by persistent problems with hyperactive and impulsive behaviour and difficulty maintaining concentration and attention on specific tasks. The conditions have a range of symptom severity from mild and only minimally impairing up to severe behavioural disruption and almost complete functional impairment. An estimated 5 to 10 percent of the population suffers from some component of attention deficit.

Conventional treatments range from behavioural therapy to neuro-stimulant medications, like methylphenidate.

Efficacy of Medical Cannabis

Currently, we lack any RCTs or higher-level scientific evidence proving efficacy of cannabis medicine in these conditions. However, strong anecdotal and case-report evidence shows cannabis benefit in patients with severe ADD/ADHD. At cannabis conferences, patient families tell stories of children who had severe behavioural symptoms that were resistant to conventional medications having remarkable responses and improvements with cannabis medicine. While ADD and ADHD are known risk factors for problematic cannabis use, mounting evidence suggests improvements in cognitive performance, hyperactivity, and impulsivity with cannabis use.

Summary of Research

Studies show that individuals with diagnosed attention disorders are more likely to use cannabis in a problematic way than individuals without these disorders.[74] This increased tendency toward substance abuse may be because individuals with attention disorders often self-medicate with cannabis after discovering relief of symptoms.

Despite very little formal evidence supporting cannabis use for ADD/ADHD treatment, a recent survey of ADHD discussion forum participants revealed that 25 percent of polled respondents felt cannabis was an effective treatment.[75] In addition, a small (thirty participants) RCT of Sativex oromucosal spray showed improved cognitive performance, hyperactivity, and impulsivity.[76] While not definitive, this study provides preliminary evidence supporting the effectiveness of cannabis in treating attention disorders. Additional larger RCTs are needed to understand the role of the ECS in individuals with attention disorders and define the exact role of cannabis in treatment.

AMYOTROPHIC LATERAL SCLEROSIS

Amyotrophic lateral sclerosis (ALS, also known as Lou Gehrig's disease) is a neurodegenerative disorder of unknown origin that typically causes gradual muscle wasting, weakness, and paralysis. It's an uncommon condition affecting approximately only four per hundred thousand individuals. There is no known cure although a recently introduced medication, edaravone, appears to slow progress of the disease through antioxidant mechanisms. Most existing treatments are for symptom relief.

Efficacy of Medical Cannabis

Many patients with ALS use cannabis with the primary goal to relieve appetite loss, pain, depression, and spasticity, and ALS is a qualifying condition for medical cannabis in Canada and in multiple US States. Though no evidence currently suggests that cannabis can alter the course of this neurodegenerative disease, emerging data show that the ECS may be involved in the pathogenesis of ALS and that cannabinoid therapy is potentially beneficial.

Summary of Research

Although no large RCTs have been conducted, a survey of a small group of ALS patients using cannabis reported that cannabis was effective at reducing symptoms of appetite loss, depression, pain, spasticity, and drooling.[77] However, a 2010 study evaluating the effect of oral THC on relief of cramps in ALS patients did not find a statistical difference between the THC treatment and placebo.[78]

Despite this lack of proven benefit, a more recent review concluded that there is a valid rationale, and enough evidence, to propose using cannabinoid compounds in the pharmacological management of ALS patients.[79] Additionally, since we know that CBD and other cannabinoids are antioxidants and that the new antioxidant ALS drug edaravone is showing promise, there is reason to believe cannabinoids may be helpful. A summary paper in the *American Journal of Hospice and Palliative Medicine* concluded that based on currently available scientific data, it's reasonable to think that cannabis might slow the progression of ALS, potentially extending life expectancy and reducing the overall burden of the disease.[80]

ALZHEIMER'S DISEASE

Alzheimer's disease is an age-related neurodegenerative condition associated with cognitive decline, wasting, and death. The hallmark of the disease is the deposition of ß-amyloid proteins in the brain, which impair neuronal function and are commonly thought to cause the neurodegenerative disease. Alzheimer's is associated with progressive neuroinflammation, cellular damage, and cell death. With the demographic shift to an older population, the prevalence of Alzheimer's disease is climbing sharply with at least 10 percent of persons over sixty-five affected and almost 40 percent of persons over ninety-five affected. A number of current pharmaceutical treatments are available to help slow down the course of the disease through attempts to improve neural communication in the brain. There is no known cure.

Efficacy of Medical Cannabis

Accumulating evidence that plant cannabinoids exert a neuroprotective effect suggests that cannabis may alleviate or slow the symptoms of neurodegenerative conditions. To date, however, only small studies have provided evidence of medical cannabis benefit in treating the symptoms of Alzheimer's disease, and studies have yet to show whether cannabinoids can alter the course of the disease.

Summary of Research

Currently, no definitive research or RCTs prove benefit of cannabis treatment in Alzheimer's disease. However, there are plausible mechanisms by which cannabinoids may be helpful. For example, in brains obtained from Alzheimer's patients, alterations in ECS components have been reported, suggesting that the system either contributes to, or is altered by, the process of Alzheimer's disease.[81]

Researchers have concluded that targeting cannabinoid receptors on neuronal cells may reduce neuroinflammation, which is a feature of Alzheimer's disease. Using non-THC cannabinoids, this treatment should be possible without causing potentially negative psychoactive side effects. Cannabinoids may offer a multi-faceted approach for the treatment of Alzheimer's disease by providing neuroprotection and reducing neuroinflammation while simultaneously supporting the brain's intrinsic repair mechanisms.[81]

A 2004 study showed that CBD exerts a combination of neuroprotective, anti-oxidative, and anti-apoptotic effects against ß-amyloid peptide toxicity in cell cultures.[82] In simple terms, this finding means that CBD appears to protect brains cells and reduces the neuronal cell death and degradation that is usually caused by build up of the Alzheimer's-related protein deposits. Subsequently, a 2006 study found that THC may reduce the amount of ß-amyloid in the brain,[83] suggesting that cannabis may potentially be helpful in Alzheimer's disease through more than one action.

In 2014, researchers discovered the mechanism by which THC likely causes this reduction.[84] They found that THC directly interacts with ß-amyloid peptide, thereby inhibiting aggregation of the harmful protein. At treatment concentrations, no toxicity was observed and the CB1 receptor was not significantly upregulated, meaning that levels of THC were not high enough to cause an increase in the number of receptors. This finding suggests a very low risk of treatment harm or dependency. These researchers concluded that THC could be a potential therapeutic treatment option for Alzheimer's disease through multiple functions and pathways. Furthermore, a 2016 open-label pilot study concluded that medical cannabis oil provided significant improvement in Alzheimer's symptoms and stated that cannabis therapy is a safe and promising treatment option.[85] Therefore, while we currently lack evidence to support widespread use of cannabis medicine in Alzheimer's disease, there appears to be significant promise, which hopefully will be validated in pending RCTs.

ANXIETY

Anxiety is a feeling of worry, fear, or distress that is often accompanied by physical symptoms of increased heart rate, tremulousness, and shortness of breath. Anxiety disorders include a wide range of conditions, from generalized low-grade background anxiety to disabling, severe, acute panic attacks. These disorders are extremely common, and up to 20 percent of the population experiences some form of reported problems with anxiety. In fact, anxiety and related disorders are the most common mental conditions affecting the North American population. Unfortunately, many of the conventional medical treatments, such as benzodiazepines, have significant health risks, including a high likelihood of developing drug tolerance and withdrawal. Therefore, they are neither particularly safe nor effective for long-term use.

Efficacy of Medical Cannabis

Canadian patients report that anxiety is one of the top three indications for which they use cannabis (the other two being chronic pain and sleep disturbance). Many patients report dissatisfaction with first-line anti-anxiety treatments, which are frequently associated with significant side effects. Outside of conventional Western medicine, cannabis has long been used as a natural alternative for those seeking treatment options for anxiety. Long-term cannabis users report reduced anxiety, increased relaxation, and relieved tension when using cannabis medicine.

Despite reported benefit by many patients, cannabis is also known to have an interesting paradoxical effect with regard to anxiety. Relief of anxiety at low doses may be offset by negative and opposite effects at higher doses. Acute anxiety and paranoia are known temporary and common side effects of high-dose, high-THC cannabis. This dosing sensitivity is important to understand when it comes to the potential benefit of using cannabis to treat anxiety. Until we have better evidence, the routine use of cannabis or prescription cannabinoid medications to treat primary anxiety or depression should be viewed with caution and generally discouraged in patients with history of co-existing psychotic disorders. A personal and family history of psychosis is considered a contraindication to cannabis despite some preliminary evidence suggesting that some cannabinoids may alleviate symptoms of existing schizophrenia. That evidence may also explain the high use of cannabis in this group of patients.

Summary of Research

A 2009 review stated that the exact role of cannabis medicine in the treatment of anxiety had yet to be determined.[86] And in fact, no large RCTs have specifically examined the role of cannabis medicine in the treatment of anxiety disorders. However, several smaller studies, before and since, have investigated this relationship. We have some evidence that cannabis is effective in managing anxiety and depression as reported in a 2006 study of HIV-positive patients. Of the patients who reported using cannabis to manage their anxiety symptoms, 93 percent cited an improvement in anxiety and 86 percent cited an improvement in depression.[87]

Other studies have focused specifically on the effects of CBD. A small double-blind, crossover clinical study in 2004 showed that a single 400 mg dose of CBD significantly decreased anxiety but also increased sedation. The findings were deemed to be preliminary and follow-up studies were suggested.[88] In 2011, another small double-blind RCT showed that 600 mg of orally-administered CBD was associated with a significant reduction in anxiety, cognitive impairment, and discomfort in patients suffering from generalized social anxiety disorder.[89] A 2018 study added to this mounting evidence of CBD efficacy, showing that CBD normalized regions of abnormal brain function in patients with psychotic illness.[90] Therefore, there seems to be significant potential for the use of medical cannabis in a range of psychiatric disorders. Since the relationship between cannabis and mental illness is complex, hopefully additional planned trials will help to further define the best use of cannabis medicine for these conditions.

ARTHRITIS, GENERAL

The term *arthritis* covers a wide range of conditions that cause joint pain, including osteoarthritis, rheumatoid arthritis, and inflammatory arthritis. Joint pain is one of the most common symptoms affecting Canadian patients, and approximately 25 percent of adults have been diagnosed with some form of arthritis. Traditional treatments are primarily pain medicines and anti-inflammatory drugs. Since rheumatoid arthritis is a specific form of arthritis caused by autoimmune disease, I have included a specific section dealing with it below, while the current section relates to more generalized joint pain.

Efficacy of Medical Cannabis

Since chronic pain is the number one reason patients choose to use cannabis, undoubtedly many Canadians are already using it to relieve pain specifically due to arthritis. According to the Canadian Arthritis Society's webpage, a large number of Canadians who choose to use medical cannabis do so to relieve arthritis pain. The society is part of a coalition urging the Canadian government to invest in medical cannabis research. Evidence for treating arthritis with cannabis goes back to the original Chinese pharmacopeia, where arthritis was one of the conditions for which cannabis treatment was listed. Today, the potential use of cannabis medicines for the treatment of arthritic pain, and potentially even of the underlying joint inflammation, is once again receiving attention.

Summary of Research

No large RCTs have yet examined cannabis efficacy in treating arthritic pain and joint inflammation, but preliminary evidence is positive. Research has already shown evidence of endocannabinoid irregularities in patients with arthritic disease. A 2014 paper showed evidence of significant upregulation of CB2 receptors in patients with rheumatoid arthritis.[91] This finding suggests that the body's cannabinoid system is involved in the process of arthritic disease in ways that we are just beginning to understand.

A preliminary paper investigating the safety, efficacy, and tolerability of cannabinoids in the treatment of rheumatoid arthritis showed significant pain reduction and suppression of disease activity.[92] More recent research in animal models shows potential efficacy of transdermal CBD for relief of arthritic joint pain,[93] and another study demonstrated that attenuation of early phase inflammation by CBD appears to prevent pain and nerve damage of osteoarthritis.[94] Ongoing research is looking to confirm reported anti-inflammatory effects of CBD in arthritic disease, and researchers are investigating whether cannabinoids could help with joint repair mechanisms in inflammatory arthritis. Future proposed trials include examining whether cannabis medicine is effective at eliminating pain and inflammation in joints after orthopedic surgery.

ARTHRITIS, RHEUMATOID

Rheumatoid arthritis is a systemic autoimmune inflammatory arthritis characterized by progressive inflammation of the synovial lining of the joint with resulting joint destruction, functional disability, significant pain, and possible systemic complications, including cardiovascular, pulmonary, and skeletal problems. It's often a cause of significant suffering and even early death in many affected patients. Conventional medical treatments are steroidal and non-steroidal anti-inflammatory medicines and newer biological therapies directed against autoimmune disease.

Efficacy of Medical Cannabis

Medical cannabis is a known analgesic as well as a known anti-inflammatory. Therefore, cannabis has attracted interest as a possible treatment for rheumatoid arthritis for many years. However, evidence is currently inadequate to either support or refute medical cannabis treatment in this condition. Health Canada currently supports the use of cannabis by patients experiencing pain associated with rheumatoid arthritis who have either not benefited from, or would not be considered to benefit from, conventional treatments.

Summary of Research

Unfortunately, no large RCTs have explored the efficacy of cannabis on rheumatoid arthritis symptoms, and a number of smaller clinical trials have shown mixed results. A double-blind RCT with fifty-eight patients with rheumatoid arthritis showed significant analgesic effect and significant suppression of disease activity following Sativex treatment as compared to placebo.[92] Less conclusively, a 2012 review of the literature examining the effects of multiple medications on the pain of rheumatoid arthritis reported that, while cannabis may provide a small benefit, the effect was likely not substantial enough to outweigh possible side effects.[95] Most recently, a 2018 review concluded that while the analgesic, anti-inflammatory, and immunomodulatory properties of cannabis suggest possible benefit, the available evidence is not yet sufficient to support widespread recommendation of cannabinoid treatment for rheumatic diseases.[96] Planned and ongoing basic science and clinical human trials will help further define the role of cannabis in the treatment of arthritic disease, and rheumatoid arthritis in particular.

ASTHMA

Asthma is a common and chronic inflammatory condition of the pulmonary airways, characterized by bronchospasm and airflow obstruction. Both genetic and environmental factors contribute to asthma, and symptoms include wheezing, coughing, and shortness of breath. Approximately 5 to 10 percent of the population suffers from asthma at some point in life. Traditional medical treatment involves anti-inflammatories and bronchodilators that are typically inhaled using puffers or nebulizers.

Efficacy of Medical Cannabis

When most people think of cannabis, they think of smoking, and smoking is obviously a potential cause of pulmonary disease. Interestingly, however, results of studies on pulmonary function in cannabis users have not shown clear evidence of harm. Some regular cannabis users have actually reported improvements in their asthma, and in fact, studies show that some measures of pulmonary function improve with cannabis use. However, caution is obviously advised as chronic smoke inhalation of any kind is linked with pulmonary inflammation and increased sputum production, so risks could offset potential benefits.

Summary of Research

To date, no large RCTs have specifically examined the use of cannabis as a treatment for asthma, and its use in this condition is considered speculative. While the exact mechanisms explaining the observed improvements of pulmonary function are not fully understood, we do know that cannabis contains bronchodilators, which open up airways. THC has long been known to be a bronchodilator,[97] with a 1975 study showing significant reversal of bronchospasm by THC in an experimental model of asthma.[98] In addition to THC, certain cannabis-prominent terpenes, such as pinene, are also known bronchodilators.

The presence of these compounds may explain the paradoxical observation of improved asthma symptoms in some cannabis smokers and the fact that certain cannabis strains relieve asthma more than others. Hopefully, studies underway will confirm effects of non-smoked, inhaled cannabinoids on asthma and pulmonary function. Newer delivery mechanisms, such as nebulizers and controlled dose inhalers, may also make cannabis therapy a reality for managing asthma. Trials investigating the role of these inhaled, non-smoked cannabinoids in the treatment of asthma and other pulmonary disorders are underway in Israel.

As a word of caution, although a 2012 study confirmed no evidence of impaired lung function even after long-term occasional cannabis use,[99] the NAS review found evidence of potential negative effects. The NAS analysis revealed a statistical association between both increased cannabis smoking and worsening respiratory symptoms, as well as possible risk of more frequent chronic bronchitis episodes with long-term cannabis smoking. Overall, they concluded that the risks of respiratory complications of cannabis smoking appear to be relatively small and far lower than those of tobacco smoking. Despite this relative safety, for both general medical use and specific use of cannabis in asthma, smoking is not recommended.

AUTISM SPECTRUM DISORDER

Autism spectrum disorder is a neurodevelopmental condition that covers a range of symptom types and severity. The condition typically causes variable degrees of difficulty with social behaviour, interactions, and communication. It usually manifests early in life with symptoms starting within the first twenty-four months. Between 1 and 2 percent of children are diagnosed with some form of autism spectrum disorder. Conventional treatments are usually a blend of behavioural modifications and pharmaceutical products, such as the antipsychotic resperidone. Conventional therapies have not been particularly effective in many cases.

Efficacy of Medical Cannabis

Initial reports on the efficacy of cannabis medicine in treating children with this disorder came from families who resorted to cannabis as a last resort after conventional treatments had failed. Some of the most compelling and remarkable cannabis success stories have been told to me by parents who were frustrated at having exhausted treatment options before trying cannabis. Time and time again, I have been told how cannabis has given life back to these children and their families.

Beyond my personal interactions with these families, significant anecdotal evidence shows that cannabis is often effective at normalizing behaviour in children with severe autism spectrum disorders. Success stories about children who return to normalized behaviour after previously requiring restraints or institutionalization are remarkable testimony to the potential power of this medicine. A Facebook group named Mothers Advocating Medical Marijuana for Autism (MAMMA) USA has over eighteen thousand followers, and its members are lobbying to get access to legal, regulated cannabis medicine for children with autism across the United States.

Summary of Research

Currently, no major RCTs have investigated the effect of cannabis medicine in autism spectrum disorder. However, preclinical studies are highly suggestive of potential benefit. Randi Hagerman, a world expert in autism spectrum disorder and other premutation neurodevelopmental disorders, is involved in research showing that defects in the ECS may play an important role in the mechanisms contributing to these disorders.[100] In addition to Hagerman's work, other research has confirmed the role of the ECS in neurodevelopmental disease.[101] Two trials are underway in Israel, and pre-publication results are showing significant benefits with various cannabis preparations, including non-psychoactive CBD. An upcoming study at the Children's Hospital of Philadelphia will be the first of its kind in the United States to examine the benefits of medical marijuana in children with autism spectrum disorder, and results are eagerly anticipated.

CANCER

Cancer is, at its most basic, a disorder of unregulated cell growth. However, the consequences of this unregulated growth and spread are well known to everyone. Cancer is the second leading cause of death in North America, just behind heart disease. Traditional treatment for cancer usually involves a combination of surgery, chemotherapy, and radiation. For patients with advanced and incurable cancer, treatment is usually palliative with an emphasis on comfort and dignity.

Efficacy of Medical Cannabis

The lifetime risk of developing some sort of cancer is almost 50 percent. Therefore, there is significant interest in anything that might cause or treat cancer. As cannabis medicine becomes legitimized, questions will inevitably arise regarding its potential efficacy in treating cancer. However, we currently have no conclusive evidence that cannabis is an anti-cancer agent or could treat established cancer. Nor do we have good evidence that cannabis use increases the risk for any cancers, with the possible exception of an association between a type of testicular cancer and frequent cannabis smoking. Though our current understanding is limited, many current studies are investigating the relationships between cannabis and cancer and the potential role of the ECS in the cancer-regulation process.

Summary of Research

No major RCTs have looked at the potential therapeutic benefit of cannabis on cancer. This lack of trials is partly explained by the many variables involved. Cannabis is not one standard medicine, and cancer includes a wide range of diseases. Additionally, cancer trials are difficult and expensive and usually involve comparing a current gold-standard (accepted and tested) treatment against a proposed new treatment. Those trials require a process of preclinical research and publication that may take decades. Much of this cannabinoid cancer research is now underway. In fact, some of this preclinical evidence suggests that cannabinoids and the ECS may play a significant role in cancer-regulation processes.[102]

Though we lack evidence for specific anti-cancer properties of cannabis in human subjects, we do have evidence of these properties for multiple phytocannabinoids and endocannabinoids in the laboratory, including in human cell lines (in vitro) and in animal models. For instance, two studies have shown that both the endocannabinoid anandamide and the phytocannabinoid cannabidiolic acid (the acid form of CBD) inhibit human breast cancer cell proliferation.[103,104]

Another cancer with promising preclinical and anecdotal evidence of anti-cancer cannabis effect is the primary brain tumour glioblastoma multiforme.[102,105,106] Studies have shown significant anti-glioblastoma effects of cannabinoids in the laboratory. Glioblastoma is the most common primary brain tumour and is usually rapidly deadly. Most Canadians know someone who has died of this disease. Within a year, both Canadian Tragically Hip singer Gord Downie and US senator John McCain recently died of this disease. While purely anecdotal, my own father is an unusually prolonged survivor of glioblastoma and was a cannabis user during his active treatment. While there is no definitive evidence that cannabis alters the course of glioblastoma, many patients with this condition use it to relieve the anorexia, nausea, and vomiting associated with glioblastoma chemotherapy.

Not only is it important to determine if cannabis can be used to treat some cancers, it's vital to look at whether cannabis use is a risk factor for cancer. The NAS review made several conclusions regarding the risks of cannabis use.[72] The authors found moderate evidence of *no* statistical association between cannabis smoking and the incidence of lung, head, and neck cancers. They also found insufficient evidence to support or refute a statistical association between cannabis and the incidence of esophageal cancer or between cannabis use and the incidence of many other cancers, including prostate cancer, cervical cancer, malignant gliomas, non-Hodgkin lymphoma, penile cancer, anal cancer, Kaposi's sarcoma, or bladder cancer. However, they reported limited evidence of a statistical association between current, frequent, or chronic cannabis smoking and non-seminoma-type testicular germ-cell tumors. It's currently unclear whether this risk is real or not. Now that cannabis use is legal and likely to be more common, Health Canada will track long-term health outcomes associated with cannabis use.

CHEMOTHERAPY-INDUCED NAUSEA AND VOMITING

A typical side effect of most chemotherapy is nausea and vomiting, known as chemotherapy-induced nausea and vomiting (CINV). This common cancer-related symptom can be so severe that it often contributes significantly to cancer-related suffering and death. If patients can't eat or keep down fluids, they are at much higher risk of death. Multiple anti-nauseant medications exist, but many have serious side effects, including significant sedation and severe constipation, and are often poorly tolerated by patients. Also, some CINV is frustratingly drug resistant.

Efficacy of Medical Cannabis

Cannabis definitively relieves the potentially severe nausea and vomiting associated with chemotherapy. In fact, it's often the only medicine to do so and often works in cases that are otherwise drug resistant.

Summary of Research

Cannabis has been recognized as an anti-nauseant for thousands of years, and more recently its use has become established among those with CINV. Though much of this early use predates published scientific studies, growing clinical evidence confirms that cannabinoids, including synthetic cannabinoids such as nabilone, significantly relieve CINV. A 2001 review of US clinical trials found that patients who had failed on standard antiemetics experienced 70 to 100 percent relief of CINV when they smoked cannabis, while those treated with THC capsules experienced 76 to 88 percent relief.[107] A subsequent review reported that, after failing standard antiemetics, patients found significant relief of CINV with smoked cannabis and moderate improvement with THC capsules.[108]

Several more recent reviews have reported similar findings. A 2008 meta-analysis of cannabis-based therapies for CINV showed that cannabinoids performed slightly better than conventional antiemetics. The review also showed that many patients preferred cannabinoids to conventional therapies because they experienced the common side effects (e.g., drowsiness, euphoria) of cannabis as beneficial during chemotherapy.[109] A 2012 Cochrane collaboration reviewed twenty-three RCTs deemed to be low- to moderate-quality and found that cannabinoids had a significant benefit compared to placebo, had a similar efficacy to conventional medicines, and were preferred by patients.[110] Most recently, a 2015 paper looked at the results of twenty-eight trials and concluded that all trials suggested a greater benefit for cannabinoids than for both standard agents and for the placebo.[111] Although future research is likely to further define potential use of additional cannabinoid preparations in the treatment of nausea and vomiting, for now the evidence is already convincing.

CROHN'S DISEASE *see Inflammatory Bowel Disease*

CONCUSSION

A concussion is a temporary loss of normal brain function that results from a brain injury, usually a blow to the head. It often results in temporary loss of consciousness. Sports-related concussions have become a common news item since repetitive head injuries are now associated with long-term and sometimes fatal brain injury. There have been very few successful treatments for concussion, and most current approaches focus on rest and avoidance of sensory stimuli while the brain recovers.

Efficacy of Medical Cannabis

Preclinical studies have demonstrated the ability of cannabinoids to aid in recovery after brain injury. Combined with anecdotal evidence, mostly from athletes, the use of cannabis and specific CBD products in professional collision sports is becoming widespread. These athletes are using cannabis products both before and after games as they are convinced of the protective and restorative properties. Additionally, a number of ex-NFL players have formed an advocacy group to support use of cannabis not only for head injury but also for chronic pain. Enough evidence of CBD's neuroprotective effects has now accumulated that both the NBA and NFL are proposing removing CBD from their lists of banned substances.

Summary of Research

Research in 1998 at the National Institutes of Health confirmed that cannabis medicine had potential neuroprotective properties,[112] and the neuroprotective and antioxidant effects of cannabis have been shown in animal models repeatedly.[113] More recently, a 2017 study showed evidence that CBD reduces neural inflammation and enhances neuroplasticity and recovery after ischemic injury in an animal model.[114] The current evidence supporting the use of cannabis medicine in the treatment and prophylaxis of head injury and concussion is currently all preclinical and from basic science research. A number of human trials are proposed, and the fact that the FDA has now approved a CBD-based medication for the treatment of seizures suggests that a new era of CBD-related human research trials is about to begin.

In the meantime, many professional athletes engaged in collision sports already take CBD due to personal belief and anecdotal evidence suggesting efficacy in both prophylaxis and treatment of traumatic injury and post-concussion syndrome. Due to increasing concern about the role of repetitive head injury in development of chronic traumatic encephalopathy, attention on the possible role of cannabinoids as neuroprotectants is sure to continue.

DIABETES

Diabetes is a disorder of glucose metabolism. It's increasingly common as obesity is a major risk factor, and it's now the seventh leading cause of death in North America. The disease has two main forms, type 1 and type 2, which relate to the body's failure to either produce or respond to the hormone insulin. Each scenario results in spikes or dips in blood sugar, which can cause dangerous results both in the short term and long term. Type 1 diabetes classically develops in younger patients and is a condition in which the body stops producing insulin. The treatment is predominantly insulin therapy. The more common type 2 diabetes is associated with obesity and is the result of the body's resistance to insulin, which the body still produces. Treatment involves diet, exercise, and a number of different potential medications.

Efficacy of Medical Cannabis

The use of cannabinoids in the treatment of diabetic disorders has been postulated for many years based on the observation that cannabis users often have more stable insulin levels and less insulin resistance than non-cannabis users.[66] Despite this association, the exact role of cannabis medicine in the treatment of diabetes remains unknown.

Summary of Research

No large RCTs have yet investigated the potential use of cannabis in treating diabetes, but some minimal good scientific evidence is suggestive of benefit. The NAS review concluded that there is limited statistical evidence to support claims that cannabis use either improves or worsens diabetes. Essentially, the authors concluded that we can't say either way. Most of the available evidence comes from preclinical studies, including a 2006 study that showed that CBD lowered the incidence of diabetes in genetically predisposed mice.[115]

We do have evidence that cannabis affects metabolic functions, some of which could be potentially detrimental to diabetic patients. Cannabis is a proven appetite stimulant, and epidemiological studies show that cannabis use is associated with higher average caloric intake levels than seen in non-users.[116] One might assume this increased intake would be bad for diabetics, but despite those associations, cannabis use has also been associated with lower body mass index, lower prevalence of obesity, and less diabetes.[117] A 2013 study also found a correlation between cannabis use and lower levels of fasting insulin, insulin resistance, and smaller waist circumference.[66] More specific evidence of direct benefit came from a small 2016 RCT that demonstrated that the cannabinoid tetrahydrocannabivarin (THCV) significantly decreased fasting plasma glucose in patients with type 2 diabetes.[118] Future trials, including planned RCTs, will hopefully better define the potential role of cannabis medicine in the treatment of diabetes.

DEPRESSION

Depression is a serious mood disorder that causes a prolonged and persistent feeling of sadness, hopelessness, and loss of interest in normal life activities. It's one of the most common mental health conditions in North America. Without treatment, symptoms can last for weeks, months, or years, and those affected are often at serious risk of adverse health events or suicide. Depression has many forms, and it often occurs in concert with other mental health conditions, such as anxiety, or serious chronic health problems, such as cancer or Parkinson's disease. Consequently, treatment can be challenging but typically includes both psychotherapy and medication.

Efficacy of Medical Cannabis

Depression is one of the more common indications for which Canadians choose to use medical cannabis. Despite this self-medication, it's not yet clear exactly how cannabinoids affect mental health or if they are an effective treatment for depression.

Summary of Research

While long-term cannabis users report reductions in anxiety, increased relaxation, and relief from tension,[86] the data on cannabis as a specific treatment for depression are mixed in their support. The NAS review found insufficient evidence to draw conclusions on the possible association between cannabis use and improvement of depressive disorders. Additionally, the authors reported that there was at least some evidence of a statistical association between cannabis use and a small increased risk of developing depressive disorders. Therefore, caution should be stressed before deciding to use cannabis medicine to treat depression. However, it should also be stressed that almost all of the analyzed data comes from research on recreational cannabis products. The efficacy of CBD and lower-THC medical cannabis products in treating depression has not been evaluated.

Other studies have investigated the mechanisms by which cannabinoids may act in the brain to influence mood disorders. Preclinical studies have shown that cannabinoids elicit antidepressant-like behaviour and activate serotonergic neurons through the medial prefrontal cortex.[119,120] Serotonin is an important neurotransmitter, and deficiencies have been linked with depression. A 2018 study confirmed that the primary antidepressant effects of CBD were related to brain serotonin levels.[120] Other mechanisms are also likely involved as there is evidence that activation of CB1 receptors has antidepressant effects in animal models.[121] Furthermore, a 2015 non-clinical study showed that increases in the endocannabinoid anandamide resulted in antidepressant and anti-anxiety activity via CB1 receptor–mediated modulation of both serotonin and norepinephrine neurotransmission.[122] All of these findings suggest that various components of the endocannabinoid system present therapeutic targets for antidepressant medications in the future.

EPILEPSY

Epilepsy is a relatively common neurological disorder marked by recurrent abnormal brain activity that typically manifests as seizures. The multiple forms of epilepsy and are often referred to as seizure disorders. They can occur at any age and may be the result of genetic predisposition, brain injury, or other disease processes. Treatment is usually one of a variety of anti-seizure medications. Unfortunately, some forms of epilepsy are drug resistant.

Efficacy of Medical Cannabis

The role of cannabis in epilepsy treatment serves as a perfect example of the dichotomy between our extensive human experience with cannabis medicine and the skeptics who say we do not have enough evidence. Cannabis has been used and reported effective as an epilepsy treatment in humans for thousands of years. In the nineteenth century, cannabinoid preparations were widely established as treatments for epilepsy. Multiple animal studies have confirmed anti-epileptic properties of cannabinoids for years. However, as recently as early 2017, most medical science reviews reported lack of data supporting cannabis as an epilepsy treatment. Now, less than two years later, a strong consensus supports cannabis treatment benefit in some forms of epilepsy. Health Canada now approves cannabis as a treatment for epilepsy when conventional treatments have proven ineffective, and based on the findings reported in the *New England Journal of Medicine* paper, the FDA and DEA approved Epidiolex, the CBD extract used in the epilepsy study. This extract is the first cannabis medicine approved in the United States, likely an important step toward full cannabis legalization south of the Canadian border.

Summary of Research

Until recently, we had conflicting evidence and opinion on the effectiveness of cannabis in treating epilepsy. For example, while both a 2001 and a 2016 study suggested that cannabis could reduce seizures, the 2017 NAS review concluded that little higher-level evidence supported its use. The 2001 study described the effects of cannabis on epileptic symptoms in humans and concluded that cannabis could be helpful in the short term for those suffering from epilepsy, but they also concluded that it was unclear what long-term effects may be.[123] The 2016 study described the experience of five Israeli pediatric epilepsy clinics treating children and adolescents diagnosed with intractable epilepsy. The study detailed the effects of CBD oil on seventy-four patients, whose ages ranged between one and eighteen years. The overall results of the study were promising, although the study was observational and non-randomized. Of the patients studied, 89 percent reported reduction in seizure frequency, and 18 percent reported a 75 to 100 percent reduction.[124]

Combined with the long historical use of cannabis as an epileptic medicine and the fairly positive results of the 2001 and 2016 studies, it came as a surprise to some that its use was not endorsed by the NAS. However, due to the statistical limitations of the prior research, the 2017 NAS review concluded that there was "limited or insufficient evidence supporting the use of cannabis in the treatment of epilepsy." These conclusions would be short lived, however. Only three months later, in May 2017, a pivotal cannabis research paper was published in the *New England Journal of Medicine*. A "Trial of Cannabidiol for Drug-Resistant Seizures in the Dravet Syndrome" was a double-blind RCT where 120 children and young adults with drug-resistant epilepsy received either CBD solution or placebo.[41] The results were conclusive: CBD resulted in a significant reduction in the frequency of seizures as compared to placebo. An accompanying editorial declared that "for cannabis and epilepsy, we have real data at last."[125] Data emerging from similar cannabis trials in other disease states will likely change the playing field just as rapidly and decisively.

FIBROMYALGIA

This disorder is characterized by widespread pain and hypersensitivity and a constellation of other symptoms, including sleep disorders, fatigue, and emotional or cognitive disturbances. The cause of fibromyalgia is thought to be multifactorial, and its diagnosis and treatment remains difficult. Fibromyalgia is common, but it's often resistant to treatment by conventional medical means.

Efficacy of Medical Cannabis

Because fibromyalgia often doesn't respond well to conventional treatments, many patients are reaching to cannabis for relief.
Extensive anecdotal and historical evidence report benefit of medical
cannabis in the treatment of fibromyalgia, although we don't have
any RCT evidence. Patients typically report most benefit from CBD oil
or high-CBD cannabis strains, and acceptance as a treatment is growing. For example, the 2012 Canadian Guidelines for the Diagnosis
and Management of Fibromyalgia state that a trial of pharmacologic
cannabinoids may be considered in patients with fibromyalgia, particularly in the setting of concomitant sleep disturbance.[126]

Summary of Research

Although no RCTs have yet examined the potential role of cannabis in this disorder, several lower-level studies have found evidence
supporting the effectiveness of cannabis in treating fibromyalgia. A
2006 study looked at the effects of prescription cannabinoids on fibromyalgia patients over a seven-month period. Participants reported a
significant decrease in pain score, a significant decrease in depression,
and a reduction in the intake of concomitant pain-relief medications,
such as opioids, antidepressants, anticonvulsants, and non-steroidal
anti-inflammatory drugs, following treatment with THC.[127]

Other studies have revealed patient-reported benefits. A 2009
cross-sectional survey of patients suffering from fibromyalgia found
that patients reported using cannabis (by smoking and/or eating) to
alleviate pain, sleep disturbance, stiffness, mood disorders, anxiety,
headaches, tiredness, morning tiredness, and digestive disturbances associated with fibromyalgia.[128] A 2011 survey of fibromyalgia
patients also showed extensive use of cannabinoids in that patient
population to relieve pain, sleep disturbance, stiffness, depression,
anxiety, and headaches.[129]

In contrast, some reviews have not been as conclusive. A 2016
Cochrane review looked for evidence to support use of cannabinoids
in the treatment of fibromyalgia.[130] The authors found only two studies large enough to be evaluated. Both of these studies examined the

efficacy of nabilone rather than plant cannabinoids. The reviewers stated that they found no convincing, unbiased, high-quality evidence suggesting that nabilone is of value in treating fibromyalgia.

More recently, however, evidence in favour of cannabis treatments has been growing. A 2017 review indicated there is enough preclinical evidence to suggest significant benefit of cannabinoids in treatment of inflammatory and neuropathic pain, including fibromyalgia.[131] Additionally, the most recent 2018 study on the efficacy of medical cannabis in fibromyalgia from Israel showed improvement of subjective symptoms in 100 percent of study participants, and 50 percent of test subjects were able to wean off all other pain medicines.[132] Ultimately, we'll need one or more rigorous RCTs to examine the potential role of cannabis medicine in the treatment of fibromyalgia before the issue is decided conclusively.

GASTROINTESTINAL ILLNESS

Gastrointestinal (GI) illness constitutes a wide range of disorders, symptoms, and problems. It covers everything from acute symptoms due to viral illness, through chronic conditions due to abnormal bowel function and chronic inflammatory conditions such as IBD. Since other sections of this part of the book cover the role of cannabis in treating the autoimmune inflammatory conditions of Crohn's disease and ulcerative colitis and the functional GI disorders of irritable bowel syndrome, this section will briefly discuss the role of cannabis in treating other GI-related symptoms. Inevitably there will be some overlap. Minor bothersome GI symptoms and complaints are common, and a multitude of over-the-counter treatments are available, from Tums to Pepto-Bismol.

Efficacy of Medical Cannabis

Cannabis has been used effectively for centuries to treat a variety of GI symptoms, including nausea and vomiting, diarrhea, and abdominal pain. The role of cannabis medicine as potential treatment for minor GI symptoms is not well defined. Since many GI symptoms are related directly to either excess or inadequate motility or peristalsis of the gut, it's likely that many of the potential cannabis effects on these symptoms are motility-related and more directly apply to the section on irritable bowel syndrome. It's also worth mentioning again that cannabis medicine is often effective at relieving symptoms at low doses but may have opposite and unintended effects at higher doses. While the effects on GI motility by cannabis may be potentially beneficial, chronic recreational cannabis use can in some situations contribute to a syndrome marked by reduced peristalsis, abdominal pain, and cyclical vomiting.

Summary of Research

Cannabis medicine has proven effective at treating several specific GI disorders (chemotherapy-induced nausea and vomiting, inflammatory bowel disease, and irritable bowel syndrome), and research on those conditions is discussed in detail in their respective summaries. As for how cannabis may affect other GI conditions, more research is needed. However, studies have shown endocannabinoid receptors widely distributed throughout the neural plexus of the GI tract,[133] which suggests a potential role of cannabis medicine for treatment of functional GI disorders. Cannabinoids are known to have a variable effect on gut motility but, in general, usually reduce peristalsis. This effect is likely why overwhelming the GI ECS with high-potency recreational cannabis contributes to cyclical vomiting and abdominal discomfort in some recreational users. These effects have not been reported with use of lower-potency medical products. Pharmaceutical modulation of the GI ECS may provide a useful therapeutic target for disorders of GI motility,[134,135] but further research is required to define this application in the future.

GLAUCOMA

Glaucoma is a multifactorial disease usually caused by increased pressure within the eye. It's characterized by progressive degeneration of the optic nerve and the death of retinal ganglion cells, ultimately leading to irreversible blindness. Increased intraocular pressure (IOP) is strongly implicated in the pathophysiology of glaucoma, although normal-pressure glaucoma can occur. Glaucoma occurs in approximately 2 percent of the population over age forty. Conventional treatments are usually eye drops that help to reduce pressure in the eye.

Efficacy of Medical Cannabis

IOP is considered the primary modifiable risk factor for the development of glaucoma. Cannabinoids, primarily THC with likely potentiating effects of CBD, are known to reduce IOP, and cannabis therefore shows promise for treating glaucoma. However, the IOP-reducing effects of smoked cannabis are short lived, and we have yet to develop cannabis therapies that alter the course of glaucoma. Therapies may improve with new delivery formulations and longer lasting cannabinoid preparations.

Summary of Research

No large RCTs have looked at the effect of medical cannabis treatment on patients with glaucoma. However, several decades of research on the effect of cannabis on IOP, beginning in the 1970s and continuing to the present day, have shown that administration of cannabinoids typically lowers IOP by up to 30 percent.[136] We also know that the ECS functions in the eye, and CB1 and CB2 receptors are also present.[137] THC appears to be the primary cannabinoid that decreases IOP, and CBD may potentiate this effect and add a degree of neuroprotection to the optic nerve.

A 2015 study suggested that the neuroprotective properties of cannabinoids combined with their ability to decrease IOP, make cannabinoids potentially useful therapeutic agents in mitigating neural cell loss in glaucoma.[138] Though smoking cannabis has been shown to reduce IOP, cannabinoid-based therapy appears to be limited by the short duration of cannabinoid action.[139] Furthermore, any cannabis-induced decreases in IOP have not yet been proven to alter the course of glaucoma. However, with current research and development into extended release formulations, it's likely that cannabis medicine will soon emerge as a viable treatment for glaucoma.

HEPATITIS AND LIVER DISEASE

Hepatitis refers to inflammation in the liver, and it has many potential causes. Hepatitis is only one form of liver disease, but viral hepatitis remains the most common liver disease in the world. Other common liver diseases include chronic cirrhosis or scarring that may result from chronic hepatitis or heavy alcohol consumption. Both hepatitis and cirrhosis can ultimately lead to progressive liver failure and death. Deaths from liver disease are increasing in North America, particularly as a result of heavy alcohol intake. Treatment for liver disease is usually withdrawal of the insulting agent, antivirals, and supportive care.

Efficacy of Medical Cannabis

Mounting evidence suggests an important role for the ECS in the pathophysiology of a multitude of diseases affecting the liver, suggesting that cannabis medicine may provide effective therapy. However, the exact mechanisms by which cannabinoids may affect the liver are not yet understood, with activation of cannabinoid receptors potentially causing both positive and negative outcomes. Further research is needed to better understand this system and develop appropriate cannabinoid therapies, although most research currently leans toward showing benefit of cannabis treatment in liver disease.

Summary of Research

Though we have evidence that the ECS functions in the liver, the CB1 and CB2 receptors appear to play potentially opposing roles. Activation of the CB1 receptors is implicated in the progression and worsening of alcoholic and metabolic fatty liver disease, liver scarring, and circulatory failure associated with cirrhosis. In contrast, stimulation of the CB2 receptors in general appears to confer beneficial effects in alcoholic fatty liver disease, hepatic inflammation, liver injury, liver regeneration, and fibrosis.[140-143] These opposing effects make predicting the effects of cannabis on liver disease difficult.

No large RCTs have investigated cannabis efficacy in liver disease, and available data are mixed. For example, a 2015 study suggested potential worsening of hepatitis C–related cirrhosis in cannabis users compared to non-users,[144] whereas a 2006 study suggested cannabis use improved symptoms, enabled patients to better tolerate anti-viral treatment, and improved virologic outcomes.[145] Despite this opposing evidence and seemingly contradictory effects of CB1 and CB2 receptor activation, the overall benefit of cannabis on liver disease appears positive.[140,142] A recent 2018 study further added evidence of potential benefit, showing that cannabis use is associated with reduced prevalence of progressive stages of alcoholic liver disease.[63] RCTs are needed to fully define the appropriate role of cannabis medicine in the treatment of liver disease.

HUNTINGTON'S DISEASE

Huntington's disease (HD) is a progressive and typically fatal genetic neurodegenerative disease. Every person who inherits the HD gene ultimately develops the disease, usually in their thirties or forties. The disease is uncommon and affects approximately five in a hundred thousand people. There is no known cure, and pharmaceutical treatments are usually directed toward symptom control and reduction of associated jerky involuntary movements.

Efficacy of Medical Cannabis

Upregulation of cannabinoid receptors has been demonstrated in a number of neurodegenerative disorders, including HD, suggesting the potential use for cannabis treatment. However, more research is needed before cannabis therapy can be recommended.

Summary of Research

Studies have shown that the ECS is involved in the pathogenesis of HD in animal models. Therefore, activation of specific targets within the ECS signaling system has been postulated as a promising therapy in HD.[146] In experimental models, specific activation of CB2 receptors has been related to a delayed progression of neurodegenerative events, particularly those related to the toxic influence of microglial cells on neuronal homeostasis.[147] Microglia are cells that are a normal part of the central nervous system and are involved in immune functions. They are known to be overactivated and responsible for neuronal injury in a number of central nervous system disorders, including HD. Control of microglia with use of cannabinoids may be a clinically promising therapy for controlling brain damage in these neurodegenerative disorders.[147] The benefits of this therapy have been confirmed in mouse models of HD, where administration of substances that increase endocannabinoid activity resulted in significant improvement of motor disturbances and neurochemical deficits.[148]

Not all research has shown such effects, however. An RCT pilot using Sativex in humans was unable to show any differences or side effects for the treatment of HD. The publication concluded that future study designs should consider higher doses, longer treatment periods, and/or alternative cannabinoid combinations.[149] Due to significant evidence of ECS alterations in neurodegenerative diseases, active research efforts are certain to continue. However, since HD is rare, research will be expensive and difficult to fund. Therefore, a change in classification of cannabis to non-Schedule I status allowing easier access to government grants will likely be required if meaningful HD-specific cannabis research is to occur in North America soon.

HIV/AIDS-RELATED ANOREXIA AND CACHEXIA

HIV infection and associated immunodeficiency syndrome was first formally identified in the early 1980s. In the almost two decades before effective antiretroviral drugs became widely available, millions of people died, mostly young men in their most productive years. A significant problem with uncontrolled HIV/AIDS is anorexia and cachexia, or wasting syndrome, which is characterized by appetite loss, weight loss, and muscle wasting. Thanks to the development of successful antiretroviral medications, full blown AIDS is now uncommon in developed countries and is becoming less common in the rest of the world. However, exisitng research on that patient population continues to inform the medical cannabis debate today.

Efficacy of Medical Cannabis

The significant potential for cannabis medicine to address HIV/AIDS-related symptoms was confirmed during the early years of HIV/AIDS research when the treatments of the time caused nausea and vomiting. Researchers discovered that cannabis use not only could improve the nausea and vomiting (research on which is discussed in the Chemotherapy-Induced Nausea and Vomiting section) but also could treat anorexia and cachexia as cannabis is an effective appetite stimulant. The ability of recreational cannabis to increase appetite has been recognized anecdotally for many years. This effect has repeatedly been reported by cannabis users both within and outside clinical settings. The "munchies" is a real clinical phenomenon, and it can be used therapeutically in medical patients. Health Canada explicitly approves the use of dried cannabis in this context when patients have not benefited from conventional treatments.

Summary of Research

Controlled laboratory studies with healthy subjects show that exposure to cannabis, whether by inhalation or oral ingestion, correlates positively with an increase in food consumption, caloric intake, and body weight.[150] A 1997 double-blind RCT with dronabinol showed significant increased appetite and weight gain in HIV patients.[151] A 2005 study further examined the effects of dronabinol and cannabis in HIV-positive cannabis smokers relative to caloric intake and mood, finding that cannabis-based therapies produced substantial increases in food intake without producing adverse effects.[152] Additionally, a 2007 study reported clinically significant muscle mass gain, overall weight gain, increased appetite and food intake, as well as improvements in mood and sleep, with both smoked cannabis and dronabinol in HIV patients.[153]

The data for use of cannabis to treat anorexia in the non-AIDS population have been mixed. Interestingly, cannabis has been shown to help increase body weight in underweight individuals but may actually help with weight loss in overweight individuals.[154] This seemingly paradoxical effect is likely related to the homeostasis role of the ECS. The exact role of cannabis in treating of anorexia and cachexia outside the original AIDS population is currently unclear, but future planned trials using specific medical cannabis products should help to provide an answer.

INFLAMMATORY AND AUTOIMMUNE CONDITIONS

When excessive inflammation occurs in the body, the result is often pain, disability, and tissue damage. Chronic inflammatory conditions are a major source of pain and suffering, and often contribute to shortened life in those affected. Autoimmune conditions cause inflammation and damage when immune cells mistakenly attack healthy tissue. They cover a very broad range of diseases, including type 1 diabetes, rheumatoid arthritis, multiple sclerosis, and Crohn's disease, which have each warranted a dedicated summary in this chapter, as well as many others, including polyneuropathy, psoriasis, lupus, and Graves' disease. Overall, there are more than eighty named conditions. An estimated 5 to 10 percent of the population is affected by some sort of chronic inflammatory autoimmune disease. Conventional treatments are steroidal and non-steroidal anti-inflammatory drugs, as well as newer biological treatments that target specific cellular inflammatory pathways.

Efficacy of Medical Cannabis

We currently lack significant evidence supporting efficacy of cannabis in these human autoimmune and inflammatory diseases, with the exception of pain and spasticity of multiple sclerosis. However, we know that inflammation is both potentially helpful and potentially harmful in the human body and that balance of inflammatory processes in our bodies is required for optimal health. We also know that the ECS plays a key role in keeping that balance. Cannabinoids have both immunomodulatory and anti-inflammatory properties and therefore have significant potential in treating autoimmune and inflammatory disease.

Summary of Research

Cannabis medicines have shown potential, although mostly unproven, benefit in the treatment of multiple inflammatory autoimmune diseases, including rheumatoid arthritis, Crohn's disease, and multiple sclerosis, research on which is discussed under those conditions. Though no large RTCs have investigated the efficacy of cannabis in treating most of these autoimmune and inflammatory diseases, significant scientific evidence shows that multiple phytocannabinoids have anti-inflammatory properties and that endocannabinoids play a role in inflammatory cell signalling pathways.[155-157]

Additional evidence suggests a likely future role for cannabinoids as combined anti-inflammatory and anti-neoplastic medication.[158] Specific research into the potential role of cannabinoid medicine in the treatment of autoimmune disease is also underway. A 2014 paper showed that cannabinoids may exert effects through epigenetic pathways, leading to potential therapies as anti-inflammatory medications in autoimmune disease.[159] A 2016 paper shows that CBD specifically can suppress transcription of pro-inflammatory genes in activated immune cells and can play a potential role in autoimmune disease.[160] Since autoimmune diseases are so common and are increasing in incidence in North America, a tremendous amount of research attention is focused on them. This research will undoubtedly involve additional trials to identify which ECS targets and cannabinoid medicines are most effective in these conditions.

INFLAMMATORY BOWEL DISEASE (CROHN'S DISEASE AND ULCERATIVE COLITIS)

Inflammatory bowel disease (IBD) refers to specific chronic inflammatory conditions of the GI tract, and they affect approximately 1 percent of the population. They are thought to be GI manifestations of autoimmune disease where the body's immune system is attacking its own tissues. The two main forms of inflammatory bowel disease are Crohn's disease and ulcerative colitis. While the two diseases share some overlap, they also have important differences. Crohn's disease is an autoimmune disorder characterized by patchy intestinal inflammation that may affect any part of the GI tract from the mouth to the anus. Ulcerative colitis is also an autoimmune inflammatory condition, but differs from Crohn's in that its intestinal manifestations are limited to the colonic mucosa. Symptoms of both are primarily GI-related, including abdominal pain, diarrhea, and weight loss, but they also include more vague systemic symptoms of malaise, anorexia, and fever. Additionally, both forms of inflammatory bowel disease are associated with possible extra-intestinal manifestations in joints, eyes, and skin. While surgical removal of the colon is a radical yet potentially effective way to eliminate most symptoms of ulcerative colitis, the diffuse nature of Crohn's disease means that there is no surgical cure.

Efficacy of Medical Cannabis

Good basic evidence suggests that cannabis is both anti-inflammatory and immunomodulatory. Animal models show that the ECS is involved in the mediation of intestinal function and inflammation, and observations of CB1 and CB2 receptor upregulation have been seen in animal models of IBD. Currently, however, no conclusive data verify that cannabis is an effective treatment for IBD other than for symptom relief. Large RCTs using measurement of serum inflammatory markers, biopsy findings, and endoscopic disease severity scores (to demonstrate objective improvement) are necessary before cannabis will be widely accepted and recommended as an IBD treatment option by the medical profession at large.

Despite the absence of rigorous evidence, numerous anecdotal reports from patients show significant improvement with the use of cannabis, particularly in Crohn's disease. As a former intestinal surgeon who managed surgical complications of inflammatory bowel disease, I had a large population of Crohn's and colitis patients. Since Crohn's disease is chronic, recurrent, and not curable by surgery, most patients and physicians try to avoid the operating room if at all possible. A number of my previous Crohn's patients chose to self-medicate with cannabis. I observed significant relief of symptoms during their disease flares and some patients even avoided surgery in a number of cases. This symptom relief and occasional remission were hard for me to understand at the time. With increasing knowledge of the role of cannabinoids and the ECS on gut function and inflammatory conditions, some of these previous anecdotal observations are starting to have a plausible underlying physiologic explanation.

Summary of Research

Numerous animal models have demonstrated a relationship between the ECS, intact GI physiology, and regulation of gut inflammation. Cannabinoid receptor activation is considered a promising therapeutic target in GI inflammatory states where there is immune activation. Researchers are also starting to look at the interplay between normal gut bacteria and the ECS as gut flora is thought to play a role in both healthy and diseased intestine.[133,161,162]

A 2011 Israeli observational study looked at the effects of canna-bis on Crohn's progression and noted a reduction in disease activity and need for surgery.[163] Additionally, a preliminary observational, open-label, prospective, single-arm trial of thirteen patients with inflammatory bowel disease reported that treatment with inhaled cannabis over a three-month period improved subjects' quality of life, caused a statistically significant increase in subjects' weight, and improved the clinical disease activity index (a standardized measure of disease activity) in patients with Crohn's disease.[164] A prospective RCT in 2013 further showed a favourable clinical response to inhaled cannabis in 90 percent of test subjects, leading to calls for further research, including RCTs.[165] This study demonstrated that a short eight-week course of THC-rich cannabis produced significant clini-cal, steroid-free benefits to ten of eleven patients with active Crohn's disease, compared with the placebo. No objective evidence of disease remission was found.

On the negative side, a 2014 study found a reduction in Crohn's symptoms with cannabis use but also found that cannabis use was a predictor of increased need for surgery.[166] As a GI surgeon, I am not surprised by these findings as increasing symptoms would lead to increased desire to self-medicate with cannabis, but ultimately the increased symptoms are likely an indicator of disease severity and need for surgery.

No large RCTs have investigated the effect of cannabis on Crohn's disease or colitis. While preliminary findings indicate therapeutic po-tential for cannabis to mitigate IBD symptoms, most human trials to date have failed to provide objective evidence of improvement on endoscopic biopsy and inflammatory marker levels. Studies showing anti-inflammatory effects of CBD, combined with anecdotal reports of cannabis-induced Crohn's remission, are spurring ongoing research in this area.

IRRITABLE BOWEL SYNDROME

Irritable bowel syndrome (IBS) is the most common functional GI disorder encountered in clinical medicine. It's a spectrum of disor-ders characterized by the presence of chronic abdominal symptoms and alterations in bowel habits. IBS is a disorder of function of the GI system, rather than a disease of its structure. Therefore, IBS is very different from IBD, which is an inflammatory condition where the underlying structure of the bowel is abnormal. While it's good news that IBS is not associated with structural GI abnormalities, it can be very frustrating for patients who undergo structural investigations, like X-ray imaging and endoscopy, often to be told "nothing is wrong" when they are in pain and are having very abnormal bowel function. A number of IBS medicines were introduced and then withdrawn from the market over the last two decades due to potentially dangerous side effects. Currently, there aren't a lot of effective medications for IBS, so a lot of attention is being focused on the potential benefit of cannabinoids.

Efficacy of Medical Cannabis

As pain is a predominant feature of IBS for many patients, cannabis has been used by patients to relieve IBS discomfort for years. IBS has variants where the GI tract works too quickly, causing diarrhea, and other variants where the bowel functions too slowly, causing constipation. As cannabis tends to slow down the GI tract, it's theoretically much more effective for treating diarrhea-predominant than constipation-predominant IBS. Further research is needed to better understand these mechanisms and refine dosing recommendations.

Summary of Research

To date, no RCTs have examined the effect of cannabinoids in treating IBS. However, some research has investigated how cannabinoids affect gut function. A 2011 trial of a cannabinoid agonist showed reduced fasting colonic motility in patients with non-constipation irritable bowel syndrome.[167] These data support the hypothesis that cannabinoid receptors play a role in controlling colonic transit and sensation in humans and deserve further study as potential mediators or therapeutic targets in lower functional GI disorders.[168] According to a 2016 systematic review of the efficacy, tolerability, and safety of cannabinoids in treating IBS and other related disorders, clinical trials returned no significant instances of cannabis curing or reversing

IBS. However, the analysis did show a clear tendency for reduced abdominal pain and increased appetite.[169] IBS is a common and bothersome condition, and the market for effective medications is large. This need will lead to commencement of planned IBS-cannabinoid medicine trials in the near future.

LIVER DISEASES *see Hepatitis and Liver Disease*

MIGRAINE HEADACHES

A migraine headache is an episodic and typically severe headache that is often associated with visual symptoms, nausea, and sensitivity to sensory stimuli. A migraine variant may have similar symptoms, but the headache may not be severe or present at all. Migraine headaches are common and occur intermittently in up to 15 percent of the population. Typically, a migraine attack will leave the sufferer unable to work or participate in normal life activities. Often, patients will need to sleep or lie down in a quiet dark room for possibly many hours until the migraine passes. Consequently, frequent migraines can be disabling. Patients are usually highly motivated to find any medication that helps, and while multiple medications are on the market for headache, many patients find their migraines are resistant to conventional drug therapies.

Efficacy of Medical Cannabis

Extensive anecdotal and historical evidence suggests benefit of cannabis in treating headaches and migraines. Currently, there is not enough evidence from well-designed clinical trials to endorse the use of cannabis for migraine headaches. However, in Canadian cannabis clinics, health care providers report many Canadians are turning to cannabis for migraine relief, particularly if standard therapies have already failed. Anecdotal reports are that these patients are finding significant relief with cannabis.

Summary of Research

Though no large RCTs have investigated cannabis efficacy, humans have been using cannabis to treat migraines and other headache disorders for thousands of years.[170] There are sufficient anecdotal and preliminary results, as well as plausible neurobiological mechanisms, to warrant properly designed clinical trials.[171] Regarding the neurobiological mechanisms, a 2012 study found differences in CB1 receptor binding in migraine sufferers, leading to suspicion that ECS imbalance may play a role in migraine headaches.[172]

Although we lack data from large RCTs, a number of recent studies have reported potential benefits of cannabis use in migraine sufferers. A 2016 retrospective chart review of 120 migraine patients who used medical cannabis on the advice of a physician showed 40 percent had significantly reduced migraine frequency and 20 percent had no further migraines.[173] An as-yet-unpublished study presented at the 2017 European Academy of Neurology meeting examined the effects of cannabis on forty-eight chronic migraine sufferers. Reports suggest they were able to demonstrate significant reduction in migraine and cluster headache frequency and severity with cannabis as compared to standard headache and migraine medicines. Further cannabis migraine trials are underway, and it's likely that cannabis medicines will become recognized as a legitimate treatment for migraine and other headache disorders soon.

MULTIPLE SCLEROSIS

Multiple sclerosis (MS) is a progressive autoimmune disease of the central nervous system that results in neurological damage due to deterioration of the protective myelin sheath around nerves. Symptoms of MS vary widely depending on the amount of nerve damage and which specific nerves are affected. Typical symptoms include numbness, weakness, pain, and muscle spasticity. MS is uncommon but not rare, with less than 0.5 percent of the Canadian population living with the disorder. There is no known cure for MS and drug treatments are typically anti-inflammatory and autoimmune medications.

Efficacy of Medical Cannabis

Although we don't have evidence that medical cannabis changes the course of MS, it's one of the conditions for which cannabis medicine has strong scientific evidence of benefit and near-universal acceptance of efficacy. Humans have been using cannabis and reporting improvement in MS symptoms for over a hundred years, and the efficacy of cannabis medicine in improving the symptoms of MS has been established for more than ten years. Improvements have been reported for relief of spasticity, chronic pain, anxiety and depression, and insomnia.

In many studies examining the effect of cannabis on MS-related symptoms, improvements were primarily seen in subjective patient reports rather than during objective measuring. Researchers speculate this lack of correlation between objective and subjective data may be explained by the complex multifactorial nature of spasticity, difficulty in objective measurements, or unexplained mechanisms of symptom relief that are difficult to quantify. Regardless of whether the improvements are subjective, objective, or both, the MS patient population is among the most vocal in its support of cannabis medicine, and it's not uncommon for these patients to say that cannabis has given them their lives back. The celebrity Montel Williams, himself an MS patient, is quite vocal in his passionate and unwavering support for cannabis medicine.

Summary of Research

Abundant high-quality evidence supports the use of cannabis in relieving patient-reported MS symptoms, a representative portion of which I'll review here. Regarding patient use of cannabis, a 2006 survey conducted in the United Kingdom reported that 68 percent of patients seeking treatment for MS had chosen to self-medicate with cannabis to alleviate their symptoms.[174]

Several studies in the early 2000s provided enough evidence to support treating MS symptoms with cannabis. These studies involved evaluation of smoked whole plant cannabis and oral cannabis extracts. This research formed the foundation that led to the eventual approval of nabiximols (balanced THC–CBD extract) for the official treatment of MS symptoms in many countries. The largest RCT of cannabis in MS, the multicentre cannabinoids in multiple sclerosis (CAMS) study with 630 patients, was published in the *Lancet* journal in 2003. This trial showed significant reduction in subjective patient-reported pain and spasticity, and it also demonstrated small but non-significant objective improvements.[175] Four additional smaller RTCs published between 2004 and 2010 confirmed that improvements with medical cannabis were seen primarily in subjective self-reports of symptoms rather than objective measurements.[176-179] An RCT in 2004 also showed significant reduction of chronic neuropathic pain and spasticity in MS patients.[180] More recently, a 2012 Canadian RCT of smoked cannabis in MS patients showed statistically significant improvement in both patient-reported pain and spasm, as well as objective measurements. The study also demonstrated significant reduction in patient scores on the visual analog pain scale.[181]

Other more recent trials have investigated the efficacy of manufactured cannabinoids and extracts. A 2011 double-blind RCT using nabiximols in refractory MS patients showed significant improvement in objective and subjective spasticity as well as secondary end points of spasm frequency and sleep disturbance. This study led to final approval of Sativex in multiple countries to treat MS.[182] A 2012 double-blind phase III RCT (the Multiple Sclerosis and Extract of Cannabis [MUSEC] trial) reported that a twelve-week treatment with an oral cannabis extract was associated with statistically significant relief in patient-reported muscle stiffness, muscle spasms, and body pain as well as statistically significant improved sleep compared to placebo in patients with stable MS.[183]

Evidence suggests that the ECS is involved in muscle tone and spasticity and shows that MS patients have deficiencies in the levels of measurable endocannabinoids, suggesting that cannabinoid treatment might alter MS progression.[184] However, a 2013 *Lancet Neurology* paper published the results of an RCT on the potential effects of THC on MS progression, and the authors found no effect on objective progression with dronabinol (synthetic THC) alone.[185] This study raises the possibility that cannabinoids other than THC, or at least a mixture of THC plus other cannabinoids, are responsible for the full therapeutic effect in MS patients. A number of new cannabis/MS research trials have been proposed and are pending, but some are currently significantly delayed due to difficulty doing research on Schedule I drugs in the United States.

NAUSEA AND VOMITTING
see *Chemotherapy-Induced Nausea and Vomitting*
AND *Gastrointestinal Illness*

OPIOID CRISIS

More than seventy-two thousand North Americans died from drug overdose last year, the majority from opioid* use. In Canada, almost five thousand opioid deaths occurred in 2017. Drug overdose deaths are now the leading cause of accidental death in North America, having overtaken motor vehicle accidents and other trauma. This epidemic is affecting all regions of the continent and all demographics. The healthcare industry has contributed to this crisis by aggressively marketing and prescribing opioid medicines for almost any painful condition. As a result, approximately 40 percent of opioid deaths are directly related to physician-authorized prescription medication.

Efficacy of Medical Cannabis

Due to the devastating effects of the opioid crisis, there is an urgent push to find safer and less addictive treatments for pain. While much of the emphasis is appropriately on non-pharmaceutical interventions, significant attention is also turning toward cannabis as a potential treatment. It's hard to ignore the fact that cannabis has caused no reported overdose deaths. Additionally, we have good evidence showing that populations with access to legal cannabis have lower rates of opioid use and that patients appear able to wean off opioids when given access to medical cannabis. However, we currently lack evidence on exactly how cannabis medicine should be used by health care providers to help their patients stop using opioids. The results of ongoing trials will hopefully clarify this situation soon.

---

*   A note on terminology: *Opiates* are a class of medicines that are derived from the naturally occurring opium poppy plant. These drugs include heroin and morphine. *Opioids* are synthetically derived medicines made in the laboratory that have actions similar to the natural opiates. These synthetic drugs include fentanyl and methadone. An intermediate class of opiate-like medicines, called semi-synthetic opioids, use synthetic alterations of natural plant compounds. These semi-synthetic drugs include oxycodone and hydrocodone. All of these medications are used primarily to treat pain, and all have a significant risk of addiction and abuse.

    The term opioid is now commonly used to refer to the entire class of medications, including the natural opiates. I use this inclusive term throughout the book, except when referring to studies that specify a particular class of these medications.

Summary of Research

A 2015 review examined the available evidence showing potential effects of CBD on different addictive behaviours in both animals and humans. They concluded that CBD appears to exert effects on various neurotransmitter systems involved in addiction. They also concluded that it likely has significant potential in treatment of various addictive disorders and also appears to be safe, non-addictive, and free of any significant side effects. These findings have spurred a number of on-going trials in both Canada and the United States.[186]

In addition to its potential use in treating addiction, mounting evidence is supporting cannabis as an alternative to conventional chronic pain medications. Studies show that patients using cannabis for pain are able to reduce pre-existing opiate use and achieve more effective control of chronic pain with cannabis than with opiates alone, and with fewer side effects.[187] A 2017 review stated that the growing body of research supports the medical use of cannabis as an adjunct or substitute for opioid use.[188] Another 2017 paper reported the results of a survey of Canadian patients using authorized medical cannabis, which showed the majority of these respondents were able to substitute cannabis for previous prescription drugs, including opioids, benzodiazepines, and anti-depressants. The primary reasons cited by patients for this substitution were fewer side effects, more safety, and better symptom management.[189]

A 2012 paper postulated mechanisms by which medical cannabis might be an adjunct to or substitute for prescription opiates in the treatment of chronic pain.[190] The paper concluded that, when used in conjunction with opiates, cannabinoids led to a greater cumulative relief of pain, resulting in reduced opiate use. Additionally, the authors suggested cannabinoids may be able to prevent tolerance development and withdrawal from opiates and may be able to rekindle opiate sensitivity after a prior dosage has become ineffective. Future research efforts are required to generate protocols that demonstrate exactly how cannabinoids should be used by health care providers to help get their patients off opioids.

PAIN

Pain may be described as an unpleasant or distressing sensation that is often caused by intense or potentially damaging stimuli. Pain is subjective, and pain is complex. Pain is not one particular thing, and what may be perceived as painful to one person may be almost undetectable to another. Pain threshold is likely partly inherited and partly learned. The perception of pain has strong cultural, emotional, and psychosocial aspects. The ongoing opioid epidemic is teaching us difficult and valuable lessons about the consequences of trying to completely free patients from pain. Total pain relief may not be worth it if the cost is not breathing.

Efficacy of Medical Cannabis

Research shows that pain is by far the most common reason patients choose to use medical cannabis, and humans have been using cannabis as part of their pain management strategy for thousands of years. Researchers are attempting to document exactly how effective cannabis is as a pain medicine in a variety of diseases, especially in situations where the sufferer has already failed other means of pain control. Despite lack of large RCTs, pain management is one of the areas for which we already have the most conclusive evidence of benefit.

However, pain is a complex and multifactorial symptom, and there are many different types of pain. Therefore, even within the pain data, the role of cannabis medicine still holds areas of uncertainty and questionable efficacy. This uncertainty is particularly true with regard to acute pain after injury or surgery. Currently, no good data verify efficacy of cannabis for management of acute pain. However, that is not the experience of many patients and health care providers. My observations of the profound opiate-sparing properties of cannabis in my own post-operative patients led to my work in the medical cannabis field. I believe data will ultimately show potential benefit of cannabis for relief of most types of pain. In the meantime, most of our pain data relate to the effects of cannabis on cancer-related pain and other chronic pain. In the section below, I examine some of the cannabis research as it pertains to these specific types of pain.

Cancer Pain

Just as pain is a complex and multi-faceted topic, so is cancer. Therefore, any discussion of cancer pain must be prefaced with the statement that each and every case will be different. However, it's true that pain and suffering are an unfortunate reality for many cancer patients and that cannabis is often used by this group. Multiple studies have shown benefit of cannabis therapy for patients dealing with moderate to severe cancer-related pain. The data are starting to reveal not only relief of pain but also of multiple additional cancer-related symptoms, such as anxiety, depression, and insomnia. The data are also starting to reveal a possible opioid-sparing effect of cannabis in this context.

Chronic Pain

More than a hundred million people are estimated to be living with chronic pain in North America.[191] Chronic pain is defined as pain lasting more than twelve weeks. Many Canadians in the senior demographic would probably laugh at this definition as pain for them has become a permanent and daily reality. I think a better definition might be persistent pain lasting more than twelve weeks that interferes with ability to enjoy life and conduct normal activities of daily living. Conventional medical therapy for chronic pain has relied heavily on opiate medicines over the last two decades. Due to the devastating results of the opioid epidemic, a major search is underway for additional effective and safer pain medicines. Management of chronic pain, particularly chronic neuropathic pain, is the area for which we have the most cannabis research data and an area that most observers, even skeptics, agree that cannabis shows efficacy.

Summary of Research

Extensive research has investigated the efficacy of cannabis in treating both cancer pain and chronic pain. Much of the work on cancer pain has investigated the benefits of cannabis as an adjunctive therapy, meaning that patients use the drug in addition to conventional medicines. In chronic pain research, a variety of studies have already examined the effect of smoked or vaporized cannabis as well as orally administered prescription cannabinoids (such as nabilone, dronabinol, and nabiximols). This research has studied various sources of chronic pain, including postoperative or traumatic pain, reflex sympathetic dystrophy, arthritis, Crohn's disease, neuropathic pain, interstitial cystitis, HIV-associated myopathy, post-polio syndrome, idiopathic inguinal pain, and chronic headaches. This list is not exhaustive and there are obviously many other causes of chronic pain. Each condition is likely to respond differently to any pain medicine, including cannabis. Below I review the cannabis research on cancer and chronic pain.

Cancer Pain

A 2010 double-blind RCT in resistant intractable cancer pain showed that nabiximols was statistically significantly effective adjunct medicine in reducing cancer pain.[192] A 2011 study, where patients used vaporized cannabis, was also encouraging, indicating that cannabis enhanced opioid therapy for pain.[193] A 2012 review further concluded that, when used in conjunction with opiates, cannabinoids led to a greater cumulative relief of pain, resulting in a reduced opiate use.[190] The study also suggested that cannabis may help prevent tolerance and withdrawal in opiate patients and that cannabis might help to make opiates effective again after a prior dosage had become ineffective due to the development of drug tolerance.

More recent research has investigated effects of manufactured cannabinoids and extracts on chronic pain. A 2017 double-blind RCT showed promising results of nabiximols as adjunctive therapy in advanced cancer patients with chronic pain that was unalleviated by optimized opioid therapy. The study found that this adjunct THC–CBD therapy was more effective than placebo on quality-of-life measurements.[194] In addition to this evidence, in a 2017 selective review of medical cannabis in cancer pain management, researchers found evidence of cancer pain reduction associated with THC use. While some studies reportedly lacked statistical power due to a limited number of study subjects, the review ultimately called for further clinical trials to establish the optimal dosage and efficacy of cannabis-based therapies.[195] Since cannabis medicine is being increasingly used by cancer patients in Canada, data is already being gathered to address some of these concerns, and future RTCs are planned.

Chronic Pain

A hallmark cannabis pain study was conducted by a Canadian team of researchers in 2010, before the current legal medical cannabis system was developed. Mark Ware, a physician and researcher at McGill University, conducted an RCT in which the efficacy of placebo was compared with three different doses of smoked cannabis. This research was one of the first randomized trials to demonstrate that cannabis could provide significant relief of chronic neuropathic pain caused by trauma or surgery.[196]

In addition to being an effective pain reliever, medical cannabis is also associated with reduced opioid use for chronic pain management. A 2016 study showed a 64 percent reduction in opioid use in chronic pain patients who started on medical cannabis.[197] A 2016 analysis of US prescription data from Medicare enrollees in states with medical access to cannabis also showed a significant reduction in the prescription of conventional pain medications, including opiates.[198] In addition, a 2017 study examined patient preferences for medical cannabis over prescription medications in chronic pain treatment. Many patients wanted to wean off prescription medication due to concerns of side effects, dependence, and tolerance. They perceived medical cannabis to have faster action, longer-lasting positive effects, and fewer side effects.[199]

Several review articles have investigated the efficacy of cannabis in treating chronic pain and have all agreed on its potential benefits. A 2009 review of eighteen double-blind RCTs concluded that evidence suggests that cannabis is moderately efficacious for treatment of chronic pain.[200] A 2015 systematic review and meta-analysis also concluded that moderate-quality evidence supported the use of cannabinoids in the treatment of chronic pain.[111] The 2017 NAS review declared there was substantial and conclusive evidence for the effectiveness of cannabis in treating chronic pain in adults.

However, despite these multiple reviews showing efficacy of cannabis for management of chronic pain, the most recent Cochrane review, published March 2018, stated that results are still inconclusive. The reviewers looked specifically at the effects of cannabis for neuropathic pain, and they based this conclusion on an absence of large rigorous trials and a presence of heterogenous results. Another systematic review paper, published in October 2018, also performed a meta-analysis of the existing cannabis pain literature and concluded that cannabis is unlikely to be an effective therapy for chronic non-cancer pain.[73] These 2018 papers both concluded that we lack enough higher-level evidence to support cannabis therapy. Once again, these conclusions highlight that while a huge amount of scientific evidence supports cannabis use in chronic pain, we still don't have sufficient level 1a or 1b evidence.

Though we await the rigorous level 1a studies, researchers have been investigating mechanisms by which cannabis works to relieve chronic pain. We know that it almost certainly works through more than one mechanism. THC appears to work primarily through CB1 receptors, both directly on nerve signalling and also on the cognitive and emotional processing of pain signals. CBD and other related cannabinoids are known to have anti-inflammatory effects that likely target different parts of the pain pathway via the CB2 receptors. A 2018 study also showed that CBD exerts effects through complex mechanisms, which include analgesic effects moderated by activation of serotonergic receptors and anxiolytic effects via activation of TRPV1 ion channels,[201] which are existing neurotransmitters and cellular signalling pathways.

Depending on the type of pain a patient is experiencing, one specific cannabinoid may have a greater impact than another. Currently, due to lack of data on what mixtures of cannabinoids are best for what type of pain, this area of cannabis medicine is also often one of trial and error. What we do know is that cannabis can have a paradoxical dose-related effect on pain, with low and moderate doses often being effective at relieving pain but higher doses sometimes increasing pain.[202] This finding was supported by a 2012 RCT that showed that low- and moderate-dose cannabis extract was more effective at relieving opioid-resistant pain then higher doses.[203] Ultimately, despite significant evidence supporting cannabis as pain relieving medicine, many unanswered questions remain. In this new era of specific cannabinoid medical preparations, we'll likely need additional RCTs proving efficacy in the treatment of different types of pain in order to settle some of this debate. Much of this needed research is either planned or underway.

PALLIATIVE CARE

Palliative care is an area of medicine that emphasizes quality of life, dignity, and relief of suffering over life extension in patients who are living with serious, life-limiting disease. With an aging demographic, by some estimates up to 80 percent of deaths will require some sort of palliative care. The ultimate cause of death in most patients with terminal disease is respiratory, often due to pneumonias or inability to clear airway secretions. Respiratory death occurs not only due to the effects of the underlying illness but also due to the sedative effects and respiration suppression resulting from multiple medications given to control pain and other distressing symptoms. Opiate and anti-anxiety medications used conventionally in palliative care often contribute significantly to sedation and respiratory death at the end of life.

Efficacy of Medical Cannabis

I believe that there are few areas of medicine for which cannabis offers more benefit than for palliative care. Medical cannabis therapy offers patient-controlled dosing and frequency of use and provides relief of multiple symptoms typically associated with serious disease. It also offers potential life extension by mitigating serious respiratory side effects of conventional medications. One of the main reasons cannabis is so safe is that it doesn't suppress breathing. Therefore, cannabis may relieve a variety of symptoms for the palliative patient, with less need for opiates or benzodiazepines and hence lower risk of respiratory depression. By not suppressing respiration, this symptom relief may also be accompanied by longer, symptom-free survival. Better life, and potentially longer life.

Cannabis use appears to be gaining ground rapidly in palliative care settings where the focus is on individual choice, autonomy, empowerment, comfort, dignity, and, most importantly, quality of life. The need for appropriate palliative care is increasing due to an aging population where the majority of deaths are caused by chronic progressive conditions.

Summary of Research

In palliative care, like many areas of cannabis medicine, research has shown improvement more often in subjective patient-reported measurements than in objective measurements. However, multiple small studies have shown the benefit of medical cannabis in meeting the goals of palliative therapy, which are relief from pain and distressing symptoms and enhancement of quality of life. Cannabis medicine provides these effects directly through its own actions and also indirectly by reducing the need for use of conventional medications, thus minimizing the sedation and respiratory depression of opiates and benzodiazepines. This indirect effect is also referred to as an opiate- or benzodiazepine-sparing property. As with other conditions, the use of cannabinoids in palliative care results in a decrease in the overall number of medications used by this patient population, which is frequently a concern for both medical and economic reasons. This decreased reliance has been confirmed in at least one study examining the effect of cannabis use on a palliative population with HIV/AIDS.[204]

In terms of direct effects, cannabis and prescription cannabinoids, such as dronabinol, nabilone, and nabiximols, have been shown repeatedly to alleviate a wide range of symptoms encountered in palliative care settings. These symptoms include intractable nausea and vomiting associated with chemotherapy or radiotherapy, anorexia and cachexia, severe intractable pain, severe depressed mood, and insomnia. Most of these data come from studies on patients with cancer or advanced HIV/AIDS. In mid-2018, an online publication from the *Annals of Palliative Medicine* summarized the data on cannabis medicine in palliative care patients.[69] This summary included analysis of multiple studies of cannabis use in over three thousand cancer patients showing significant improvement in the control of multiple symptoms, including pain, sleep disorders, fatigue, anxiety and depression, and nausea and vomiting. The study found that while only 19 percent of patients reported good quality of life prior to cannabis treatment, 70 percent reported good quality of life at six months after cannabis therapy.

Despite the strong evidence supporting the use of cannabis in palliative care, skeptics remain. As recently as February 2018, the College of Family Physicians of Canada published recommendations stating that they "recommend against use of medical cannabinoids as first- or second-line therapy for palliative pain owing to limited benefits and high risk of harms (strong recommendation)."[205] This recommendation was almost entirely based on the fact that no large RCTs were available for rigorous meta-analysis, considered a lack of data, and the frequent occurrence of temporary intoxication by recreational cannabis, considered a high risk of harms. I don't mind going on record stating that those were ridiculous assertions with regard to the likelihood of producing patient harms. Cannabis as a palliative treatment for cancer patients is a well-tolerated, effective, and safe option to help patients cope with the cancer-related symptoms.[71]

Unfortunately, some palliative patients have had trouble accessing cannabis medicine. One study suggested the primary barrier for those using cannabis in palliative care has been the difficulty with accessing and administering the medicine, rather than any complications resulting from the medicine itself.[206] Given the safety of cannabis and its known positive effects as an antiemetic, an appetite stimulant, a sedative, and a pain reliever, its effectiveness in palliative care is obvious to most patients. Institutional and health care provider support is often more challenging. This issue should improve with education, evolution of cannabis legislation, and familiarity with cannabis research data. In fact, a recent study published in the online version of the *Journal of Clinical Oncology* showed that 80 percent of cancer specialists in the United States now discuss medical cannabis with their patients, 67 percent believe it's a helpful pain treatment, and 65 percent believe cannabis is equally effective to, or more effective than, standard medications for nausea and vomiting.[70]

Mounting evidence clearly supports cannabis as a therapeutic agent to relieve multiple symptoms in the palliative care population.

Combined with decreasing social stigma, this evidence will inevitably result in increasing cannabis therapy in these patients.

PARKINSON'S DISEASE

Parkinson's disease is a degenerative neurologic disorder marked by tremors, stiffness, and progressive difficulty with movement. The disease typically starts later in life and appears to be related to loss of nerve cells that produce the neurotransmitter dopamine, which is required for normal motor function. There is no medical cure for Parkinson's disease. Primary treatments are aimed at replacing dopamine and controlling symptoms.

Efficacy of Medical Cannabis

Clinical trials concerning the efficacy of cannabis in treating Parkinson's disease have been inconclusive. Cannabis is therefore not yet recommended for treating Parkinson's disease, though preclinical trials have shown promising results and further research will hopefully elucidate more information.

Summary of Research

Reports of using cannabis to treat Parkinson's disease go back to the late 1800s. Despite this evidence, no large RCTs have investigated cannabis efficacy. However, some of the evidence suggesting possible benefit to Parkinson's patients comes from animal models, including a 2002 paper that showed that stimulation of endocannabinoid receptors reduced dyskinesia (difficulty with movement) in a primate model of Parkinson's disease.[17] Additionally, preclinical trials looking at the potential impact of cannabinoids on movement disorders in general have been promising and warrant further investigation.[207] More recently, a 2014 preliminary double-blind RCT examined the effects of CBD on Parkinson's disease and showed improved quality of life but no improved motor symptoms.[208]

Much of the human cannabis research in this area has been observational, including several surveys completed by patients suffering from Parkinson's disease who self-medicated with cannabis. In a 2017 survey, the average patient rating of the efficacy of cannabis in treating Parkinson's symptoms was 6.4 on a scale from 0 to 7, and the majority of the six hundred participants reported being able to reduce their intake of prescription medication since beginning cannabis treatment.[209] In further testament, the results of an earlier 2017 study investigating the experience of Parkinson's patients with medical cannabis found that symptoms improved in the initial stages of treatment without any major adverse side effects.[210]

The most recent review of cannabis and Parkinson's disease concluded that results from available clinical studies were inconclusive due to limitations including small sample size, lack of standardized outcome measures, and expectancy bias (the influence of researcher expectations on likely outcomes).[211] The authors stressed that well-designed studies involving larger numbers of patients, objective biological measures, and specific clinical outcome measures are needed to clarify the effectiveness of cannabis-based therapies in Parkinson's disease. Researchers in the United States are poised to start cannabis trials in Parkinson's disease, but these studies will likely need to wait until anticipated rescheduling of cannabis occurs.

POST-TRAUMATIC STRESS DISORDER

Post-traumatic stress disorder (PTSD) is a psychiatric condition marked by recurrent and often disabling strong and unpleasant thoughts and feelings, usually triggered by memories of a significantly traumatic event. PTSD is at epidemic proportions in North America after decades of almost constant military conflict. A Canadian study suggested that one in six veterans report PTSD symptoms,[212] and studies from the US Department of Veterans Affairs show that, on average, twenty veterans die every day from suicide.[213] Estimates are that the majority of these ex-soldiers were suffering from PTSD and that the condition afflicts 10 to 30 percent of former veterans who served in active combat situations.

Another major contributor to PTSD is sexual assault, a significant problem in many of Canada's communities. Canada has a particularly high rate of PTSD, and one recent study found Canada with the highest rate of PTSD out of twenty-four Western countries studied.[214] Traditional treatments for PTSD haven't been particularly successful, and sufferers of PTSD have often resorted to conventional medications, such as opiates and benzodiazepines, that have contributed to the prescription drug crisis.

Efficacy of Medical Cannabis

Currently, no conclusive scientific data support the use of cannabis in PTSD, although the available evidence suggests benefit. Regardless of scientific evidence, what is clear is that many patients with PTSD choose to use cannabis. Active soldiers and veterans, for instance, have self-medicated with cannabis for decades. In fact, due to early experimental evidence, PTSD is now one of the approved conditions for medical cannabis in many US states. While the current lack of high-quality trials makes any definitive conclusions about the role of cannabis in treating PTSD impossible, there is hope for more definitive answers soon. An RCT has begun in Canada, and a major FDA-approved RCT is nearing completion in the United States.

Summary of Research

Though no RCTs have yet been completed, research shows that cannabis may alleviate PTSD symptoms in a number of ways. These potential mechanisms include the ability of cannabis to produce mild dissociation from a linear sense of time, allowing users to escape the subconscious replay of traumatic events in their minds. Studies have also shown that both THC and CBD can help eliminate aversive memories, which are often the triggers for the recurring anxiety and suffering experience by PTSD sufferers.[215] Two other 2014 studies showed cannabis benefit, including significant reduction of PTSD symptoms on the Clinically Administered PTSD Scale (CAPS),[216] and a significant improvement in global symptom severity, sleep quality, frequency of nightmares, and PTSD hyperarousal.[217]

Despite a lack of conclusive evidence regarding benefits or mechanisms of action, self-medication rates among PTSD sufferers is common, particularly in military veterans. A 2016 survey of 120 Canadian Armed Forces veterans who reported PTSD showed that approximately 50 percent of this group used cannabis, a rate markedly higher than that of the general population.[218] In the United

States, 41 percent of veterans who use cannabis state that they do so for medical purposes, again a rate significantly higher than that of the general population.[219] A 2014 study also found increased rates of coping-oriented cannabis use and greater frequency of cannabis use among medical users with high PTSD scores compared with low PTSD scores. The need for sleep improvement was the primary indication for cannabis use.[220]

The future of cannabis research for PTSD is promising. A 2017 review concluded there is enough evidence to suggest that therapeutic cannabis will be a useful future treatment in PTSD,[221] and more rigorous studies are underway. In 2014, using funds from cannabis licensing and taxation, a multimillion-dollar grant was awarded in Colorado to fund a multi-institutional FDA-approved RCT of cannabis in veterans. The US study is nearing completion and should provide valuable data to help determine whether cannabis benefits PTSD. A Canadian RCT through a partnership between the University of British Columbia and the LP Tilray is also underway.

SCHIZOPHRENIA

Schizophrenia is a chronic and usually disabling psychiatric condition. Hallmarks of the disease are distorted thoughts, hallucinations, and feelings of fright and paranoia. The condition typically starts in the late teens or early adult years and often results in affected individuals being unable to participate in normal life activities. Schizophrenia affects approximately 1 percent of the population, and conventional medical treatments are primarily antipsychotic medications.

Efficacy of Medical Cannabis

The debate around cannabis and schizophrenia is complicated and paradoxical. While we have epidemiologic evidence linking cannabis use to an increased risk of psychotic mental illness in genetically predisposed individuals, emerging evidence suggests that some cannabinoids may improve cognition and thinking in individuals with existing schizophrenia. This recent evidence may explain the observation that many patients with schizophrenia choose to self-medicate with cannabis. The complex relationship between cannabis and schizophrenia strongly suggests that the ECS may be involved in normal cognitive processing and perception of reality. These ideas have stimulated a large amount of cannabis research in this area. Data guiding appropriate use of cannabinoid medicine in psychotic mental illness are likely to emerge in the coming years.

Summary of Research.

Though we have little official data on using medical cannabis to treat schizophrenia, the following studies demonstrate the complex and somewhat paradoxical nature of our current knowledge. A 2017 study from Israel showed that THC exposure in genetically predisposed mice increases the risk of developing a psychotic disorder.[222] These results support established evidence showing a link between schizophrenia and cannabis use in teenagers and young adults.[223] A 2014 study also provides evidence that a genetic predisposition to schizophrenia is associated with increased use of cannabis, independent of the development of schizophrenia symptoms.[224] This evidence strongly suggests some sort of poorly understood link between the genetic underpinnings of psychotic mental illness and cannabis.

What is unclear currently is to what degree cannabis is a risk factor for developing schizophrenia versus a potentially useful therapy in treating schizophrenia. A recent RCT has confirmed that CBD normalizes brain function in regions associated with psychotic illness.[90] Evidence also suggests that CBD improves cognitive function and reduces psychotic symptoms in patients with schizophrenia.[225] These findings have generated a lot of excitement in the neuroscience and psychiatric communities and will spur new research trials in the coming years.

SKIN DISORDERS

The largest organ in the body by both weight and surface area is the skin. The skin is also exposed to the external environment and its many potential harms and irritants. Consequently, skin disease is very common. Estimates are that almost one third of the population suffers from some sort of skin disease, ranging from acne through psoriasis and serious skin cancers. An almost unlimited number of prescription and non-prescription medications are currently available for the management of skin disease, but chronic skin disease is often relatively resistant to pharmaceutical therapy, and new effective treatments are always being sought. Consequently, there is a lot of excitement about the potential benefit of cannabis medicine.

Efficacy of Medical Cannabis

Research on how cannabis could help with diseases of the skin is in its early stages, but we do know that the ECS is present in the skin and cannabinoid treatments show therapeutic promise. Topical cannabinoids are increasingly used by dermatology patients for a range of disorders. However, the acceptance of these over-the-counter products by the general public has far outpaced scientific investigation into their safety and efficacy. Since the skincare portion alone of the beauty industry is worth an estimated $130 billion annually worldwide, this area of cannabinoid medicine is likely to attract a lot of research and business attention.

Summary of Research

The cutaneous ECS likely has a crucial role in regulating skin cell proliferation, survival, and differentiation, as well as normal dermatological immune function, according to a 2009 review of the cannabis literature with regard to skin disease.[226] The authors postulated that normal ECS balance is required for skin health and that disruption of this system might allow multiple pathological conditions and diseases of the skin to develop. Therefore, the ECS and phytocannabinoids have been identified as major potential therapeutic targets for the treatment of dermatologic disease.[227]

The types of conditions that cannabis may help treat range from skin-related pain to psoriasis and acne. Research in 2003 revealed that the combination of topical cannabinoids and opiates was far more effective at relieving skin-related pain in an animal model than opiates alone.[228] A 2007 study showed that cannabinoids inhibit keratinocyte proliferation and therefore suggested a potential role for cannabinoids in psoriasis treatment.[229] More recently, in 2014, research showed significant suppression of sebaceous gland function and inflammation using CBD, suggesting potential significant benefit in acne and inflammatory skin conditions.[230] A 2016 preclinical study supported this finding, concluding that CBD showed potential benefit in acne treatment.[231] Those researchers also found that certain cannabinoids, including cannabigerol, had potential to treat dry-skin syndrome. Due to huge economic incentives, a lot of active research has begun in an attempt to develop and prove efficacy of a multitude of cannabinoid skin preparations.

SLEEP DISORDERS

Sleep disorders are defined as difficulties with the sleep process that interfere with either the quality, quantity, or timing of sleep. In most cases, if severe, they result in difficulty with normal enjoyment of life or functioning during the day. Almost 40 percent of the adult population suffers from some degree of disrupted sleep, and sleep disorders contribute to significant suffering in the general population. The most common sleep disorders are insomnia (difficulty initiating or maintaining sleep) and sleep apnea (intermittent interrupted breathing). A large number of conventional pharmaceutical treatments are already available for insomnia, although many of these have significant side effects. Current treatment for sleep apnea is predominantly use of continuous positive airway pressure (CPAP) machines.

Efficacy of Medical Cannabis

Difficulty sleeping is one of the top three conditions for which Canadians choose to use cannabis medicine. THC is a known sedative, and for many years it has been widely observed anecdotally as an effective treatment for insomnia. Despite this common use, the scientific evidence supporting cannabis use in sleep disorders is mixed. Although increasing evidence is suggesting benefit for sleep apnea, the use of cannabis for this condition remains controversial. The theoretical risk for any sedative medicine is that it might exacerbate sleep-related apneic episodes in patients with obstructive sleep apnea. With cannabis, this theoretical risk appears to be offset by improvements in overall sleep mechanics and the fact that, while it may be sedating, cannabis medicine doesn't appear to influence respiratory drive. Studies investigating cannabinoids and obstructive sleep apnea have suggested that synthetic THC cannabinoids, such as nabilone and dronabinol, may have short-term benefit for sleep apnea due to their modulatory effects on serotonin-mediated apneas. Few studies have examined the effect of cannabis plant extracts specifically on either insomnia or sleep apnea.

Summary of Research

While few rigorous RCTs have been conducted specifically on effects of cannabis and sleep disorders, numerous studies examining the impact of cannabinoids on sleep have been done within the context of chronic pain conditions.[232] Many studies have pointed to the benefit of cannabis in the treatment of sleep disturbances associated not only with chronic pain but also with other conditions, including HIV/AIDS-related anorexia and cachexia, MS, ALS, spinal cord injury, rheumatoid arthritis, fibromyalgia, IBS, PTSD, and advanced cancer.

Most of the literature to date has studied the effects of THC on sleep since THC is sedating. As long ago as 1973, studies showed that THC reduces time to sleep in healthy individuals.[233] However, research has also shown significant sleep disturbances and vivid dreams as a consequence of cannabis withdrawal.[234] A 1981 trial of epilepsy patients showed potential efficacy of CBD in treating sleep disturbance,[235] raising the possibility that cannabinoids other than THC may be helpful. A 2010 trial once again confirmed efficacy of THC in treating insomnia associated with fibromyalgia.[236] A 2017 review of the literature on the effects of cannabinoids on sleep disorders reported that, although THC decreases sleep latency, THC alone could impair sleep quality over the long term.[232] However, it also stated that nabilone may reduce nightmares associated with PTSD and may improve sleep in patients with chronic pain. Most recently, a 2018 fully-blinded RCT (phase 2 of the pharmacotherapy of apnea by cannabimimetic enhancement, or PACE, trial) of dronabinol treatment efficacy in people with moderate or severe obstructive sleep apnea showed significant improvements in a number of sleep parameters as compared to placebo.[237]

While CBD is more associated with mental alertness, the positive effect of CBD on many illnesses that affect sleep quality may make it a legitimate sleep agent as well. The 2017 review of the cannabis sleep literature concluded that CBD may have therapeutic potential for insomnia treatment and that while THC decreases sleep latency, it might impair sleep quality long term.[232] The review further stated that CBD may hold promise for REM sleep behaviour disorders and excessive daytime sleepiness. The authors concluded that research on cannabis and sleep is still in its infancy, that current evidence is mixed, and that additional controlled and longitudinal research is critical. The demand for safe, effective sleep medicine is strong, and the fact that Canadians are already using it for this purpose essentially guarantees that research will occur.

SPINAL CORD INJURY

A spinal cord injury is an injury to any part of the spinal cord or to the major nerves within the spinal canal below the end of the cord. Injury is usually the result of an accident or trauma and typically causes permanent changes in strength, sensation, and other body functions below the site of the injury. The injury may be partial, where some function may exist below the injury, or it may be complete, resulting in total paralysis. High spinal cord injuries at or above levels related to breathing control may be immediately or ultimately fatal. There are an estimated one hundred thousand patients living with spinal cord injuries in Canada. There is no cure for spinal cord injury and current treatments are only supportive.

Efficacy of Medical Cannabis

To date, there is no good evidence that cannabis medicine can influence the course of spinal cord injuries. However, self-reported regular use of medical cannabis is significantly higher in patients with spinal cord injuries than in the general population. This use is mostly to relieve symptoms of pain and spasm.[238]

Summary of Research

Like in so many areas of cannabis medicine, large RCTs are lacking. However, multiple small studies show benefit, and subjective improvement in these patients is often dramatic. Patients appear to know of these possible benefits, and studies suggest large numbers of spinal cord injured patients continue to use cannabis to relieve symptoms. Cannabis use in the spinal cord injury population has been common for many years, and a 1974 survey documented improvements in subjective pain and spasticity in this population.[239] In 1982, further research confirmed the benefit of cannabis in relieving symptoms of spasticity related to spinal cord injury.[240] Multiple subsequent studies have confirmed relief of spasticity and pain with cannabis use in spinal cord injury.[241-243]

Much like the cannabis data for other better-studied conditions, however, the data on cannabis for relief of pain and spasm in spinal cord injured patients appear to show benefit primarily on subjective rather than objective measurements. Consequently, a 2010 review found equivocal data on efficacy of cannabis for relief of pain and spasms after spinal cord injury.[244] Due to the lack of large RCTs examining the effectiveness of cannabis on spasticity after spinal cord injury, the NAS review concluded that there is not enough evidence to conclude that cannabis medicine is effective for treating spasticity in this population.[72]

Despite this lack of higher-level conclusive evidence, recent research is suggesting exciting new possibilities. Preclinical data from 2012 suggest that the endocannabinoids acting through CB1 and CB2 receptors are part of an early neuroprotective response triggered after spinal cord injury that may be involved in healing and recovery after an incomplete lesion.[245] Therefore, the scientific community is interested in the potential of cannabinoids to actually treat spinal cord injury rather than just relieve symptoms. This idea remains theoretical, however, and extensive further research would be needed for validation.

TOURETTE'S SYNDROME

Tourette's syndrome is a neuropsychiatric condition characterized by multiple involuntary vocal and motor manifestations, called tics. It typically has onset in childhood or adolescence, and many sufferers have associated neuropsychiatric comorbidities, including ADHD, obsessive compulsive disorder, sleep issues, depression, and migraines.[246] The specific manifestations of Tourette's, such as tics and vocalizations, usually go away as the patient ages into adulthood. It's estimated to affect 0.5 percent of children, and treatments are primarily behavioural therapy and psychiatric medications.

Efficacy of Medical Cannabis

Overall, there is no clear consensus that cannabis definitely does or does not help patients with Tourette's syndrome. Since most Tourette's patients are young and the manifestations usually go away as patients age, evidence must show benefit before potential harms of any medication are justified. Anecdotal evidence and case reports do suggest improvement of symptoms associated with Tourette's syndrome with cannabis therapy. While older clinical trials failed to prove evidence of this, newer studies are beginning to show promising results.

Summary of Research

The NAS review concluded that despite a lack of RCT data, case reports suggest that cannabis does reduce the frequency and severity of Tourette's tics.[72] Large RCTs are needed to validate results of these smaller studies before cannabis is a widely accepted treatment in these difficult situations. Some researchers have hypothesized that the therapeutic effects of cannabis in Tourette's might be due to the anxiety-reducing properties of cannabis rather than to a specific anti-tic effect. Therefore, CBD may be the predominant cannabinoid responsible for beneficial effects in these patients.

Recent studies have continued to provide evidence of cannabis benefit in treating Tourette's syndrome. In a 2017 study, researchers examined the case of two young male German patients who suffered from severe, treatment-resistant Tourette's.[247] After sustained cannabis treatment at a very low dose, both patients had significant symptom improvement. In another recent study, clinicians evaluated the effectiveness and tolerability of cannabis in nineteen adults with Tourette's syndrome.[248] Over the course of the study, tic-related scores decreased by 60 percent, and eighteen of the nineteen participants showed significant improvement. Multiple case reports continue to emerge showing efficacy of cannabis in the management of otherwise treatment-resistant Tourette's syndrome.[249] Pending research trials will hopefully validate this use.

TRAUMATIC BRAIN INJURY

Traumatic brain injury is defined as temporary or permanent disruption of normal brain function caused by a blow, strike, or penetrating injury to the head by an external force. A concussion is also a common form of traumatic brain injury and has been discussed separately. While sports injuries and motor vehicle accidents are common causes, falls in the elderly cause most incidences of traumatic brain injury each year in North America. Almost two million traumatic brain injuries occur each year. Conventional treatments are mostly limited to supportive care but include epileptic medicines for patients with seizures.

Efficacy of Medical Cannabis

Mounting evidence suggests that endocannabinoids, phytocannabinoids, and some synthetic cannabinoids have neuroprotective effects following brain injury, suggesting that cannabis therapy may help treat traumatic brain injuries. Research on the efficacy of cannabis is in early stages, but we're beginning to understand the mechanisms by which cannabinoids may protect and even help repair neural tissue following injury.

Summary of Research

We know that the ECS is present throughout the central nervous system and appears to have an extensive role in nervous system development, homeostasis, normal function, and nervous system disease.[250] While research on the direct effects of cannabis on post-concussion syndrome in humans is lacking, as discussed in the Concussion section, preclinical findings have shown that cannabis offers therapeutic benefits following brain injury. Studies have shown that CBD may exert neuroprotective and neuroregenerative properties by activating serotonin receptors, causing increased cerebral blood flow.[251]

Cannabinoid-receptor agonists, including phytocannabionods, may also be helpful as they inhibit production of inflammatory compounds that are factors in causing neuronal damage. Studies show that formation of the endocannabinoids anandamide and 2-AG is enhanced after brain injury, and evidence suggests that these compounds can reduce secondary neuronal damage. Some plant and synthetic cannabinoids that don't bind directly to cannabinoid receptors have also been shown to be neuroprotective, possibly through their direct effects on other neurotransmitter systems and/or as direct antioxidants.[252]

The ECS has also been shown to play an important role in reparative mechanisms and inflammation under pathological situations by controlling some mechanisms that are shared with other neuroprotective pathways. Brain edema, neurological impairment, diffuse axonal injury, and microglial activation are all influenced by CB1 and CB2 receptor action.[253]

Numerous studies on experimental models of brain toxicity, neuroinflammation, and trauma support the hypothesis that the ECS is part of the brain's compensatory and repair mechanisms. These effects are likely mediated by cannabinoid receptor pathways that are linked to survival and repair of nerve cells. The levels of 2-AG, possibly the most abundant endocannabinoid, are significantly elevated after traumatic brain injury. When 2-AG is administered to mice with traumatic brain injury there is a decrease in brain edema, inflammation, and area of dead tissue. There is also improved clinical recovery. Due to the observed inhibition of excitatory neural transmission, inhibition of the brain's inflammatory response, and reduction of blood vessel spasm, cannabis medicines that mimic the endocannabinoids anandamide and 2-AG should be considered as candidates for cannabis-based drugs for traumatic brain injury treatment.[254] There is a lot of excitement about the potential of cannabinoid medicine in this area, and phase II trials on the effect of CBD preparations in traumatic brain injury are already underway.

ULCERATIVE COLITIS *see Inflammatory Bowel Disease*

CHAPTER 9

ACCESSING AND PRESCRIBING MEDICAL CANNABIS

Since the Cannabis Act became law in Canada on October 17, 2018, many people have been asking what the difference is between medical and recreational cannabis. Despite the fact that both products come from the same plant, there are important differences. The products are different, and the intentions of the users are different. Recreational cannabis products are usually high in THC and are deliberately used to maximize psychoactive and euphoric side effects, while medical cannabis products are typically lower in THC and are used to relieve symptoms with as little impairment as possible. These different desired outcomes have resulted not only in the development of separate medical and recreational product lines but also in separation between medical patients and recreational consumers.

Prior to recreational legalization, there was some question about whether a separate medical cannabis stream would continue after passage of the Cannabis Act. We now know that the answer to this question is a clear and definitive yes. As discussed in Chapter 3, Health Canada has declared that the ACMPR regulations will remain in place for at least five years and that the majority of phytocannabinoid products will be kept as prescription-only products. The result is that, despite recreational legalization, Canadian medical cannabis patients will continue to require the authorization of a health care provider to obtain specific medical cannabis products. Therefore, in this next section I discuss how patients can access medical cannabis through conventional medical channels and how health care providers can assist them in this pursuit.

ACCESSING MEDICAL CANNABIS THROUGH CONVENTIONAL MEDICAL CHANNELS

The journey to become an official medical cannabis patient usually starts with a visit to a health care provider. In the majority of Canadian provinces and territories, a standard health care visit with a licensed physician is required in order to obtain a medical document authorizing cannabis. In Ontario, Manitoba, and Nova Scotia, patients may also see a licensed nurse practitioner. These health care providers are the only individuals who are legally allowed to issue cannabis-authorizing medical documents in Canada. The signed medical document allows patients to buy legal, quality-controlled medical cannabis products from Canadian LPs.

Prior to Canada's formal medical cannabis legislation, many Canadian patients chose to self-medicate with cannabis, and some continue to do so now. However, the self-medication approach is not considered the safest, most reliable, or most effective way of using cannabis as medicine. Access through a licensed health care provider allows cannabis authorization to occur within the context of a complete health evaluation. Not only will health care providers be able to assess whether cannabis is safe and appropriate for individual patients, but they will also be able to recommend particular formulations of cannabis for specific conditions. Additionally, they will help patients structure a dosing regimen and provide ongoing medical advice concerning cannabis-based therapy.

Medical Cannabis and Health Care Providers

Cannabis medicine is unique in a few important ways that may affect how some health care providers approach cannabis therapy. First, its reintroduction came not through the conventional medical establishment or from the pharmaceutical industry but instead came from public and patient demand for access. The result is that legalization of medical cannabis was not supported by large phased drug trials (including the RCTs discussed in previous chapters). Therefore, for health care professionals to embrace medical cannabis, they need to be willing to view evidence beyond large RCTs and to think outside the box. Not all health care providers are willing or able to do so. Second, cannabis is really the only legal compound that has legitimate recreational and medical properties. Since some providers still don't agree with the legalization of recreational cannabis, it's challenging for them to consider cannabis as medicine. Finally, very few licensed health care providers who are practicing today received any medical cannabis education at all. While more cannabis educational material is becoming available every day, the process of cannabis self-education can be laborious and more of a challenge than many providers are willing to tackle. This need for education combined with the caveats and qualifications that accompany virtually every statement made concerning medical cannabis leaves many health care providers hesitant. However, the challenge remains that, by federal regulation, Canadians can access medical cannabis only through conventional medical channels. In other words, patients must see a physician or nurse practitioner to obtain a medical cannabis authorization.

This access requirement creates a dilemma, and it's one against which some medical professional groups have tried to push back. Medical cannabis is still new to most practicing physicians and, as a group, physicians are typically cautious and quite slow to accept change. All physicians are different and must exercise their own discretion when offering therapy to patients. Therefore, a physician's approach to medical cannabis will likely depend on prior education, exposure, experience, and culture. In Canada, physicians and other medical practitioners are still polarized with regard to medical cannabis. A growing group of physicians recognizes the incredible safety profile of cannabis and its amazing therapeutic potential. However, there are also physicians on the opposite side of the debate who grew up in an anti-cannabis culture and were educated that cannabis is never good. Because it typically takes fifteen to twenty years to change widespread established practice habit in medicine, the attitude of many of these physicians may not change during their practice lifetimes. Some Canadian physicians remain in the middle ground between the already convinced and the hardened skeptics. For these physicians, the reversal of stigma with legalization, continuing education, and the emergence of positive new study data will likely satisfy their remaining questions.

Cannabis Clinics

Due to decades of prohibition, medical cannabis is often in high demand. Currently, thousands of patients across Canada are interested in accessing medical cannabis for a variety of health problems. Because many Canadian health care providers still feel unprepared and undereducated to see medical cannabis patients, most Canadian medical cannabis patients see providers at dedicated cannabis clinics. A lot of demand has therefore been placed on these clinics staffed by physicians with expertise in cannabis medicine. The overall lack of health care providers in Canada who are currently comfortable with cannabis medicine has created a backlog of patients, which results in high volume at these clinics and presents a challenge in meeting the needs of every new and continuing patient.

In order for cannabis clinics to meet growing patient demand, patients often initially consult with a clinical extender before seeing a physician. As with other areas of health care, cannabis clinics often employ a variety of healthcare professionals, all of whom work as a team under the direct supervision of a licensed physician. Among these professionals are registered nurses, physician assistants, clinical assistants, and medical office assistants, collectively called clinical extenders. Using these extenders helps clinics handle the high demand for medical cannabis and provide more face-to-face interaction and education to every patient. As the title suggests, these individuals work as extensions of the physician, and they are supervised by the physician. They are trained healthcare professionals and medical cannabis experts capable of broadening the scope of the physician's practice.

Health Insurance Coverage

Increasingly, Canadian health insurance plans are starting to cover the costs of cannabis medicine, but only if accessed through conventional medical channels. For many patients, cannabis may already be covered by their health insurance policies if they have extended benefits. Coverage depends on the company they work for and on the health insurance provider's policy. Canadian businesses are responding quickly to the changing cannabis regulations and updating their insurance policies accordingly. More and more insurance providers are following suit. To find out whether an individual company covers medical cannabis costs, patients should speak with their employers, usually human resources staff, or their health insurance providers.

MEDICAL DOCUMENT

To legally purchase medical cannabis from Canadian LPs, medical cannabis patients need an authorizing medical document from their health care provider. This requirement hasn't changed with recreational legalization and implementation of the new Cannabis Act. Until cannabis products are given drug identification numbers (DINs) by Health Canada, the document generated by the health care provider is considered an authorization, called a medical document, rather than a true prescription. However, because the medical document authorization is essentially a prescription, and will officially become a true prescription for any cannabis products that are issued DINs, I use the terms interchangeably throughout the text unless discussing the particulars of the medical document itself.

An official medical cannabis document has several important features. First, it requires the signature of a licensed physician or alternatively, in Ontario, Manitoba, or Nova Scotia, a nurse practitioner. This signature makes the document legally equivalent to a prescription. Second, it must specify the amount of cannabis in grams per day that the patient is permitted to order from one of Canada's LPs. Third, it must specify the time period for which the medical document is valid. Finally, it must contain patient-specific and provider-specific information that is similar to what is required on a conventional prescription. However, it's essential for both patients and prescribers to understand that the medical document does not currently allow the provider to dictate dosing schedules, product types, or intake methods. Let's take a closer look at these stipulations as well as these other important considerations that work alongside the medical document.

Grams per Day

When health care providers write medical cannabis documents, they are required to specify a quantity of cannabis in grams per day (written, for example, as 1 g/day) that a patient is permitted to order from one of Canada's LPs. This grams-per-day specification is *not* a recommended dosing schedule, and the provider is *not* advising the patient to use this amount of cannabis each day. The grams-per-day quantity simply specifies the amount of dried cannabis or equivalent that a patient is legally allowed to purchase. The grams-per-day amount translates into a monthly supply of cannabis from an LP, which should be consumed based on the provider's dosing recommendation.

It's important to realize that it takes significantly more grams of dried cannabis material to make a much smaller amount of cannabis oils or gelcaps. Therefore, even if a patient's initial cannabis needs are small, the lowest grams-per-day authorization that allows purchase of any oral cannabis product is usually 1 g/day. A medical document with less than 1 g/day will usually not allow patients to order oil products from most Canadian LPs. The grams-per-day authorization is based on grams of dried cannabis flower or the equivalent. Exact dosing conversion between dried cannabis flower and oils made from cannabis extracts is complex and depends on many variables, including how many grams of dried plant product are required to produce a set amount of oil. Most Canadian LPs have a conversion chart available. For example, an LP oil might have an equivalency factor of 1 g dried cannabis to every 5 mL of cannabis oil. In that case, each 100 mL bottle of that LP's oil would be equivalent to 20 g of dried cannabis authorization.

International studies show an average use between 0.5 and 3 g/day of dried cannabis or equivalent by medical cannabis patients.[255-257] Recent data from Canadian LPs showed an average of 2 g/day.[258] Patients rarely require authorizations for more than 5 g/day, but exceptions do exist. In order to minimize unnecessary patient expense and avoid over-prescription of product, I usually recommend start-ing with 1 g/day medical document authorization for cannabis-naive patients. Once again, it's important to remember that the 1 g/day authorization is *not* the recommended starting dose. It's the amount of product the patient is allowed to order, and this authorization is strictly required under ACMPR law on the medical document. For a recreational cannabis user, 1 g of dried cannabis would typically be rolled into two to three cannabis cigarettes, or joints. This quantity would not be considered a huge daily dose for an experienced canna-bis user. However, 1 g of dried cannabis is very different than the 1 g/day equivalent of THC oil. For high-THC oil, 1 g/day is a huge dose that is potentially dangerous and could cause serious side effects, such as hyperemesis or acute psychosis. It's important that patients understand the difference between the amount they are allowed to order, as specified on the medical document, and the amount of medicine the health care provider recommends they start taking (for example, a few drops of oil under the tongue).

Typically, in contrast to the conservative recommendations for cannabis-naive patients, I recommend starting medical patients who are experienced cannabis users at 3 g/day. That amount is usually ad-equate for most medical patients, and it's rare for a patient to require authorization for more than 5 g/day. Many cannabis clinics have a policy that requires consultation with a specialty pain physician and/ or an addiction specialist prior to authorizing more than 5 g/day. The 5 g/day limit is also in line with the ACMPR and the new Cannabis Act, which specifies a maximum personal possession limit for med-ical cannabis of 150 g, equating to a thirty-day supply of 5 g/day. I'll provide more guidance on the grams-per-day authorization in the Assessing Prospective Patients section below.

Time Period
Along with grams-per-day authorizations, official medical documents must specify a time period for which they are valid. The maximum time period allowed, and the one most commonly issued, is one year. Under the ACMPR, the allowed period of use was dated from the moment the medical document was issued—not from the moment

of registration with an LP or from the moment medical cannabis product was actually received in the mail. This caused problems for some patients who experienced long delays between the day they were issued their medical documents and the day that their medicine arrived. This timing restriction has changed under the new Cannabis Act, and now the effective date of the medical document begins when a registration document is issued by an LP. Experienced cannabis clinics are familiar with all current regulations and can help ensure that patients access cannabis medicine in a timely manner.

Additional Recommendations

The revised ACMPR still doesn't give health care providers control, via the medical document, of many important details pertaining to their patients' use of medical cannabis. It doesn't allow them to dictate exactly what cannabis products patients purchase or to define specific doses or use patterns. Therefore, health care providers usually provide additional written recommendations separately from the medical document. Ultimately, each patient will decide if they will follow their providers' recommendations. Most Canadian medical colleges recommend that providers indicate specifically whether a patient should use a CBD, THC, or balanced THC–CBD product. Some also recommend that health care providers make set dosing recommendations. Although this information must currently be written separate from the authorizing medical document, eventually providers will likely be able to make more specific product and dosing recommendations as they do with conventional pharmaceuticals. It's up to each provider to understand and follow the guidelines and standards of their own provincial or territorial licensing bodies.

Currently, a provider's recommendation for specific medical cannabis products does not limit what kind of cannabis products patients are legally allowed to purchase from LPs. A patient who is given a 2 g/day authorization with a recommendation for CBD oil could use that medical document to purchase a 2 g/day allotment of THC gelcaps or dried cannabis flower. Although providers may be given the ability to specify and dictate cannabis product purchases in the future, no such regulations currently exist. This will likely need to change if cannabis medicine is to be fully embraced within the conventional medical community. Most health care providers are not comfortable with patients being allowed to purchase a different prescription medicine than the one prescribed. Regulations aside, most patients do follow their providers' advice. They understand that following these recommendations will provide the best likelihood of a favourable medical result with limited side effects.

Using the Medical Document

The medical cannabis document typically stays with the medical clinic that issued it, and the clinic sends it securely to the LP. This process is similar to filling a prescription at a pharmacy, where the original prescription document stays on file with the pharmacist. LPs can authorize purchase of cannabis only when they receive a medical document via secure digital transmission or electronic fax from the health care provider who issued it. LPs are obligated by ACMPR rules under the Cannabis Act to accept medical documents only from providers whose signatures they have verified in advance. Hence, a medical document is primarily an electronic document, which is valid to LPs only when faxed securely by the prescribing provider.

Medical cannabis patients should be aware of a few additional facts related to the medical document. A medical document authorizes patients to purchase medical cannabis from an LP, as discussed above, or to register with Health Canada to produce their own cannabis or designate someone to produce it for them. The medical document alone does not authorize patients to possess or share cannabis in public beyond what is allowed for any adult Canadian. In order to legally possess more than the recreationally allowed limit of cannabis in public, a medical patient must be able to produce either the registration document from the LP, the registration certificate from Health Canada for personal or designated medical production, or a registration certificate issued by Health Canada for medical possession only. The possession-only certificate is new under the 2018 Cannabis Act and was made available to meet the needs of Canadian medical cannabis patients who choose to use cannabis products purchased online or from regional authorized cannabis stores.

Patients are allowed to obtain a copy of their medical document for their own records, for insurance purposes, to show to employers to help demonstrate the legitimacy of medical cannabis use at work, or to initiate the grow-at-home licence. Until recently, patients were not allowed to copy their medical documents and send them to any LPs themselves. This restriction limited the options for obtaining medical cannabis in Canada to the original ACMPR model of LPs and potentially to some of the newer authorized provincial outlets. However, a number of Canadian pharmacy chains have recently announced their intention to enter the medical cannabis market and have applied to Health Canada for the relevant licences. In September 2018, Shoppers Drug Mart was granted approval by Health Canada for cannabis licensing. As of April 2019, patients now have the ability to mail, fax, or drop off their medical documents in select pharmacies in Alberta and Ontario. Therefore, in the not-too-distant future, it is likely that patients across Canada will be able to send or take medical documents to their local pharmacy to obtain cannabis medicine, just as they would take a prescription in for other conventional prescription medicines.

ASSESSING PROSPECTIVE PATIENTS

The most important decision a health care provider makes with regard to authorizing medical cannabis is whether cannabis medicine is suitable for a particular patient and whether the medical benefits of cannabis outweigh potential risks. The other primary task of the provider is to make initial recommendations regarding which cannabis products should be used and in what dose and frequency. Whether a provider chooses to prescribe cannabis to a patient, and how many grams per day are authorized, will be determined by the factors pertaining to that individual patient and also by provider-specific factors. For instance, the experience of a patient seeing a health care provider whose current practice revolves entirely around the prescription of medical cannabis will likely be very different from that of a patient seeing a cannabis-naive provider or non-cannabis specialist.

No set standards or guidelines for medical cannabis practice currently exist, so variability in recommendations from one provider to another are more likely to occur than in standardized areas of medicine, such as diabetes care. Evolving practice standards and more strict dosing guidelines will develop as cannabis research progresses. Ultimately, the decision to recommend any particular medical therapy should come only after the provider and the individual patient review the risks and benefits of the proposed treatment. While scientific generalizations and population statistics can guide therapy, each individual is unique, and what applies to one patient may not apply to another with similar symptoms. Below, I review the factors that influence the decision to prescribe or not prescribe cannabis medicine to a patient.

Indications for Prescription

Usually, one of the first things a health care provider will want to know is the specific symptom or disease condition that a patient is suffering from. The approach to an otherwise healthy person with insomnia is very different from the strategy used in a cancer patient who wants pain relief without drowsiness or sedation. From a discussion of the presenting problem or conditions, the provider will ask further questions. Health care providers need to know what treatments have been tried in the past and how effective or ineffective they were.

Most health care providers in Canada whose practices are oriented around the prescription of cannabis are comfortable prescribing for a wide variety of common symptoms and conditions. This practice is currently supported by Health Canada, which lists a wide range of conditions for which cannabis therapy is indicated, including "any disabling condition for which standard treatments have failed." However, most of the more rigorous research in cannabis has shown conclusive efficacy in a more restricted set of conditions. Depending on whose guidelines are being used, the list of conditions varies, but there is general agreement that good evidence supports use of medical cannabis in chronic pain, chemotherapy-induced nausea and vomiting, pain and spasticity of multiple sclerosis, anorexia and cachexia of HIV/AIDS, drug-resistant pediatric epilepsy, and pain and suffering in palliative and oncology patients. However, since there is no consensus in the medical community currently regarding the cannabis literature, some physicians and some provincial regulatory bodies are comfortable recommending use of medical cannabis only for an even further restricted set of conditions. Again, the set of conditions varies from one source to another. The Health Canada list is different from the National Academies list, which is different from the College of Family Physicians list. The decision-making approach of an individual health care provider will be influenced by many factors, including the guidelines and standards of their medical societies and provincial licensing bodies.

For Canadian patients seeking symptom relief with medical cannabis, the variety of cannabis guidelines for health care providers doesn't seem to have much influence. Studies show that the majority of Canadians use medical cannabis for one of three common conditions: chronic pain, insomnia, and anxiety.[40,259] Only the first of these is on the list for which most health care providers agree we have enough evidence of cannabis benefit. For both insomnia and anxiety, rigorous cannabis research is lacking, but patient demand for treating those conditions with medical cannabis is not decreasing. Luckily for patients, most experienced cannabis health care providers include a much longer list of health conditions for which they feel there is reasonable evidence of cannabis efficacy. As mentioned above, this approach is endorsed by Health Canada, which approves cannabis for the treatment of any debilitating condition that has failed conventional therapy. Therefore, patients should be truthful with their health care providers about their medical cannabis needs since many are willing to consider cannabis authorization as long as potential benefits outweigh risks.

Medical History

In order to make an accurate medical diagnosis and develop an informed treatment plan, an understanding of the patient and their medical history is required. Cannabis medicine in this respect is no different than any other area of medicine. The more information a patient can supply to the health care provider, such as history of illness, current and past medications, and surgeries, the more specific the provider can be in recommending how to use cannabis and which particular cannabinoids might be most beneficial. Furthermore, most Colleges of Physicians and Surgeons throughout Canada—those regulatory bodies that establish the parameters for a physician's practice—specify that medical cannabis should be prescribed only after conventional treatment options have been tried and proven ineffective. Providers are more likely to recommend cannabis treatment if they have a full understanding of the patient and their condition and what other treatments have been tried previously.

For patients, honesty is important in any medical setting as a health care provider can accurately and appropriately give advice only when given a full and truthful history of prior experience with cannabis (and any other substances or medications). Accurate information is essential as it's used to adjust treatment recommendations to a patient's particular needs. If a patient reports chronically using, for instance, 3 g/day of recreational cannabis with no relief of symptoms, the provider can use this information to adjust the medical document authorization to suit those needs. If that patient instead pretends to be cannabis naive, the provider will almost always issue an initial prescription for a low daily allotment that, because of the patient's developed tolerance, may not allow for effective therapy.

Prescribing Guidelines

One of the potentially frustrating situations for health care providers who are just starting to learn about cannabis medicine is the lack of established prescribing and dosing guidelines. Most prescription drugs come with a package insert or formulary advice that helps limit and guide treatment decisions, but this information is not currently available with cannabis medicine. I've already discussed the reasons behind why basic drug dosing trials have not been performed with cannabis, but the result is that we are left with prescribing and dosing decisions based on a mixture of science, experience, and common sense. Some providers are okay with this reality, and others are not. With time and ongoing research, more refined guidelines and protocols will emerge.

For this discussion, you'll notice that I've addressed *prescribing* and *dosing* separately. As mentioned above, the prescribing part of cannabis medicine involves completing and signing the medical document authorization. Because the medical document regulations allow health care providers to set only the grams-per-day authorization and the time period allowed, the provider makes dosing recommendations separately from the medical document. Therefore, I'll address these two actions separately as well. Currently, at the most basic level in cannabis medicine, only the medical document is required. Product and dosing recommendations are strongly recommended, but they are not actually legally required. As long as patients have been granted a signed medical document stating the required patient and provider data, plus grams per day and time limit, they are able to make medical cannabis purchases. Since generation of the medical document is the regulated and required part of the process, I discuss that first before continuing with an approach to the more specific dosing guidelines. Generating the medical document is relatively simple and requires a relatively brief discussion, but dosing warrants a more detailed discussion, as you will see in the dosing section later.

So first, let's look at my basic approach for starting patients on cannabis medicine by determining their suitability for medical cannabis treatment and the appropriate relative grams-per-day allotment. This approach can be used by health care providers new to cannabis medicine and is based on existing evidence and the known areas for which the two main cannabinoids, THC and CBD, have demonstrated efficacy. It's also based on the observation that experienced cannabis users develop a tolerance for THC effects in particular and can usually start at higher doses. The chart on the facing page shows a very basic approach to authorizing grams per day and recommending products to new medical cannabis patients. It's in no way a definitive guideline.

As recommended in the chart, a low starting dose and a correspondingly low daily grams-per-day limit authorization is important for cannabis-naive patients in order to proceed slowly and carefully with therapy. In the chart, I suggest that a 0.5 to 1 g/day authorization is appropriate for cannabis-naive patients. Even that much cannabis may sound excessive for someone new to cannabis, especially if the 1 g/day authorization is confused with recommended dose. It's worth

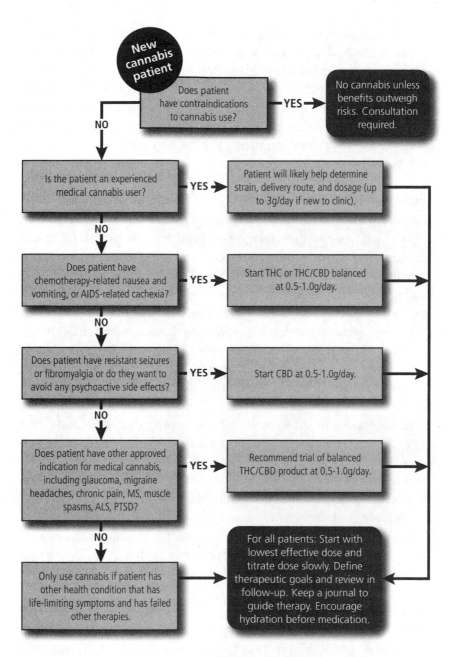

Figure 1: Flow chart showing a basic approach to authorzing grams per day and recommending products to new medical cannabis patients, giving consideration to contraindications, patient experience with cannabis, and condition being treated.

again emphasizing that the grams-per-day authorization allows purchase of the equivalent grams per day of dried cannabis flower. It's not the recommended daily dose. Due to extraction techniques and other variables involved in the production of cannabis oils, 1 g/day is the minimum required by many LPs in order for a patient to order medical cannabis oil or gelcaps. Since most cannabis-naive patients prefer to start with oral cannabis, I think an easy-to-remember 1 g/day authorization is appropriate for most new patients.

Follow Up

For any patient with active, ongoing medical problems, close and regular follow-up with a health care provider is essential. Cannabis medicine is ultimately just medicine, and regular follow-up with a provider is required and should be based on medical necessity. Follow up is particularly important for patients actively adjusting their doses, having side effects, or experiencing additional health concerns. While most general medical follow-up appointments are booked based on medical need, some provinces have set mandatory follow-up care for patients receiving medical cannabis authorizations. For instance, cannabis patients living in Alberta are required to see a health care provider every three months, even if they are healthy and stable. This mandate was set by the College of Physicians and Surgeons of Alberta as a measure to maintain some oversight and caution upon introduction of cannabis medicine (which the college did not favour). While enforced mandatory medical follow-up is potentially a waste of both time and money, for the new cannabis patient it's also a potential opportunity to review therapy and ask questions about dosing, frequency, and alternative cannabis products. For patients with ongoing active medical issues, follow-up appointments should not depend on arbitrary fixed intervals and should always be based on medical need.

DOSING GUIDELINES

Although the chart in the previous section, outlining an approach to the new cannabis patient, can be used as a guide to initial therapy, you may notice that it does not include dosing recommendations. Cannabis science is not yet advanced enough to provide firm dosing and titration guidelines, and dosing recommendations are not required on the medical document. Multiple variables currently make generation of strict cannabis dosing recommendations difficult. These include the fact that multiple strains and potencies of cannabis are available, and each strain may have varying concentrations of multiple cannabis compounds. However, using observations gathered from hundreds of thousands of medical cannabis patients and the known concentrations of the primary cannabinoids in regulated cannabis, we are able to make some slightly more scientific recommendations. With time and investment into cannabis research, more scientific trials should give health care providers the information they need to make more accurate and specific dosing and frequency recommendations.

Until standardized dosing guidelines are developed, health care providers and patients will continue to work together to develop individualized dosing regimens. Providers will provide guidance throughout this process, but each patient will help determine the best regimen through a slow and careful adjustment of cannabis dose and frequency. While the lack of strict dosing recommendations may be frustrating for some patients, self-directed adjustment gives control and flexibility, allowing patients active participation in their own health care. Patients can adjust and fine tune their medication schedules until they arrive at a regimen that perfectly meets their individual needs. Patients typically like having control of their own health and often enjoy the process of adjusting their medication. Therefore, this process is usually seen by most patients as a positive and is usually not a burden. For many, this personalized medicine approach is a welcome change from the traditionally rigid and somewhat inflexible aspects of conventional Western medicine. Below, I present a safe and careful approach to dosing in the individual medical cannabis patient.

Start Low and Go Slow

Pending development of refined and accurate dosing guidelines, a key tenet of cannabis medicine can be expressed in the message, "Start low and go slow." In other words, start at the lowest effective dose and titrate dose and frequency slowly upward according to the general guidelines outlined below. If undesirable side effects occur, then decrease the dose or try a medical cannabis product with a different THC:CBD ratio, remembering that most side effects of cannabis are the result of THC.

While the start-low, go-slow mantra is widely accepted by most experienced cannabis health care providers, it's considered too loose by many medical scientists who were trained on the fixed dosing paradigm of conventional pharmaceuticals. However, the start-low, go-slow advice is not just cautious common sense, it's based on actual evidence. The first piece of evidence is that cannabis is known, through experience and many smaller studies, to produce beneficial effects at very low doses (so-called micro-dosing). Therefore, a very low dose is sometimes all that is required to control symptoms, and in fact higher doses are sometimes less effective or have opposite effects. The second piece of evidence is that cannabis is known to be incredibly safe, and starting at a very low dose allows a large dosing range for patients to try without the significant safety concerns that are common with many other drugs. The start-low, go-slow recommendation is also based on trying to avoid unpleasant side effects and on the principle that cannabis therapy is highly individualized. Therefore, slow titration is often required to find the most effective dose. Remember, the number one goal of medical cannabis therapy is to relieve symptoms without impairment or bothersome side effects. This outcome is most likely to be achieved by starting with a very low dose. While the start-low, go-slow approach has proven to be safe and effective, the concept of a very low dose is subjective, and I discuss more specific dosing recommendations below.

Calculating Dosage

In order to provide more specific dosing recommendations, it's important to start with some basic assumptions and calculations based on traditional cannabis use. These simple calculations can be used to determine basic dosing units. We know that a typical recreational cannabis cigarette, or joint, contains approximately 0.5 g, or 500 mg, of cannabis. With an average potency of 20 percent THC in modern dried cannabis, we then know that a joint contains approximately 100 mg THC. The average joint will last ten to twenty inhalations, or puffs, and a single inhalation will therefore typically deliver 5 to 10 mg of THC. Therefore, we can derive the basic dosing unit for cannabinoid medicine in milligrams of cannabinoids. This estimate is only crude, as there are many variables, but it allows us to at least start talking about cannabinoid dosing in more precise terms. Ultimately, when the market has introduced metered dose inhalers and other set-dose delivery mechanisms, health care providers will be able to recommend precise dose measurements. With the lack of precision of current products and intake methods, multiple factors will affect the actual dose received by the patient, including depth of inhalation, absorption, and individual metabolism.

However, using the calculations outlined above, we are left with a basic single starting dose of 5 to 10 mg of THC. While 10 mg of inhaled THC has different effects and is metabolized differently than an equivalent ingested dose, the industry-standard recreational cannabis edible also usually contains 10 mg of THC per serving (a serving could be one gummy bear or cookie, for example). While these calculations are made specifically for THC, since it's the most common primary cannabinoid and the chemical for which most recreational product is made available, the same calculations could be made for any cannabinoid for which there are known percentages in the dried product. This 10 mg THC standard for cannabis edibles was developed based on real-world experience of observed effects on recreational cannabis consumers. These consumers are looking for a recreational effect. For a novice medical cannabis user, one standard cannabis edible or one big inhalation from a joint could produce slight impairment or negative side effects. Even though these effects will typically be mild and self-limited, the recommended starting dose for medical patients is lower than the standard single recreational dose. Due to lack of data, the original starting doses for THC are usually applied to the CBD-predominant and other medical cannabis products as well. Since we know that most cannabis side effects are related to THC and that many medical cannabis products have little to no THC, starting dose recommendations discussed below are even less likely to produce impairment or side effects.

As mentioned above, cannabis studies have shown that medical cannabis is often effective at very low doses,[260] typically much lower than the dose required for a recreational effect. As previously mentioned, cannabis can also have paradoxical or opposite effects at very high doses. Therefore, taking this knowledge and what we know of standard recreational doses, a safe and more scientific recommendation than "start low and go slow" is to start a patient on 2.5 mg of the chosen cannabinoid twice daily. This dosage can be applied most easily to oral cannabis products with known concentrations of cannabinoids, as the milligram dose corresponds to a set volume of cannabis oil. Using THC as an example, a 2.5 mg dose is only a quarter of a standard single recreational dose, a dose so low that chance of toxicity or side effects even with pure THC is incredibly low. A comparison to another well-known standard single serving of a recreational intoxicant would be alcohol. If one beer is a standard single serving, a quarter beer would have almost no potential for significant toxicity or harm.

Considerations Beyond Simple Dosing

Other important considerations in making cannabis-use recommendations include an understanding of the function and effect of different ratios of the primary phytocannabinoids. The two best-studied phytocannabinoids are THC and CBD, and as discussed in Part II, they have very different effects when used in isolation, but also different effects when used in varying ratios. Many Canadian LPs recognize this fact and produce a range of products with either more or less of one cannabinoid in relation to the other.

Almost all negative cannabis side effects come from THC, which is the only significantly intoxicating psychoactive compound in cannabis. Though psychoactive, THC also has powerful medicinal properties, and in fact its psychoactivity is likely responsible for many of its positive therapeutic effects. Whether the psychoactive effects are regarded as good or bad depends on dose and the presence or absence of impairment of function. Psychoactivity is the result of interaction with CB1 receptors in the brain. Too much THC can produce psychoactivity to the point of impairment. A lower dose of THC will often produce enough psychoactivity to be helpful without being harmful. While CBD is currently attracting the most attention as a therapeutic cannabinoid, it's important to remember that THC is a powerful and effective medicine in its own right. Additionally, evidence is accumulating that CBD seems to work better in the presence of some THC rather than as CBD alone. For this reason, most available high-CBD medical cannabis products contain at least a small amount of THC.

Unless patients have a symptom or disease for which specific THC therapy has been proven efficacious, I recommend that new patients who are naive to cannabis use either a high-CBD product or a more balanced CBD and THC product. This strategy will usually minimize unpleasant side effects and reduce the risk of intoxication and impairment. As mentioned previously, CBD tends to mitigate against THC side effects. Studies show therapeutic benefit, in most patients, with relatively low-THC products, so my initial recommendation is to start with a THC percentage of 10 percent or less. Some provincial guidelines recommend that THC percentage be written on the medical document, although this is not currently required by federal law.

When considering dosing suggestions, we generally apply the same recommendations to high-CBD products as we do for balanced products or high-THC products. It's safe to use the same guidelines since they were generated primarily with the intention of avoiding THC side effects. The higher-CBD products have less concern for unpleasant side effects, and evidence suggests that they have a very wide safe-dosing range over which positive effects are seen. If a patient is started on a high-CBD product and they do well, it can be continued. Ultimately, a therapeutic trial is often necessary to find the THC:CBD ratio that works best for the individual patient. If the therapeutic trial determines that a patient's symptoms are more responsive to THC, then the THC concentration can be slowly titrated upward as most patients will develop tolerance to the potential THC side effects over time.

However, like any area of medicine, each patient is different. Some patients do well with high CBD, some do better with high

THC, and others do best with a balanced THC–CBD product. It's also important to recognize that one product alone might not relieve all symptoms. Some patients will do well on a high-CBD product in the day for chronic pain but will require a higher-THC product at night to help them sleep. It's often a process of slow adjustment based on a patient response that requires a diary and journal to review therapy. Both a motivated patient and health care provider are necessary, but as mentioned above, many patients enjoy this approach to personalized medicine.

Dosing Recommendations by Delivery Method

Most new medical cannabis patients who have no experience with recreational cannabis prefer to use cannabis medicine the same way they take other medicines. Since most conventional medicine is taken orally, that method is what most new medical cannabis patients are requesting. In Canada, medical cannabis products currently available for oral delivery include oils, gelcaps, and a spray for under the tongue. Conventional tablet formulations will be available soon, and additional liquid medications and edible or chewable medications will likely eventually be allowed.

I'll emphasize that orally ingested cannabis is absorbed and metabolized differently from inhaled cannabis and often has delayed onset and prolonged effects. This different action is important since the experience of ingesting too much cannabis, particularly high-THC cannabis, can be very unpleasant and prolonged. Therefore, for oral ingestion, it's particularly important to start with the lowest possible dose (for example, one drop of oil or one gelcap) and to increase the dose slowly. The following sections detail dosing guidelines for the most common intake methods, oral ingestion and inhalation. (Note that I discuss available products in detail in Part IV.)

Dosing for Oral Ingestion

Although a variety of new oral medical cannabis products are likely going to be introduced in Canada soon, under the revised ACMPR rules under which we are still working, only edible cannabis oils and gelcaps containing oils are currently available from Canadian LPs.

These products are made by infusing edible food oils (like coconut oil) with cannabis extracts. They are designed to be ingested orally. Therefore, information that we have based on use of existing edible cannabis products, like those available in US states where recreational cannabis is legal, can help generate basic dosing guidelines. Even though most of these products are not currently available in Canada and are made for the recreational market, they are orally ingested cannabis products, so understanding their use can be helpful.

As outlined above, the industry-standard dose per cannabis edible is 10 mg of active cannabinoid. This standard evolved around THC specifically and 10 mg THC is the amount typically found in one cannabis gummy bear, cookie, or chocolate square. As this amount of THC contains more medicine than is often required to produce a therapeutic effect and enough to produce potential negative side effects, I recommend starting with a quarter to a half of standard edible dose. That would give us a basic starting dose of 2.5 mg to 5 mg of oral cannabis product. Since cannabis edibles are not currently legally available in Canada, this guideline requires converting the recommended dose in milligrams into an oil-based dose in millilitres.

Medical cannabis oil bottles are usually labelled with milligrams of cannabinoid per millilitre of oil. The recommended dose of 2.5 to 5 mg of cannabinoid typically converts to one or two drops, or approximately 0.1 mL, of LP-available oil. I usually recommend a starting dose of one to two drops under the tongue once to twice per day. If a patient reports no effect from this initial trial over a few days, then I recommend increasing the dose by one to two drops (0.1 mL) every two to three days. If the patient then reports symptom relief, that dose should be maintained. If the patient reports negative side effects, then the dose should be reduced. If patients are unable to find a dose that relieves symptoms, and particularly if they have no relief but do have side effects, a different cannabis product should be tried with the help of their providers. This regimen is slow but safe and requires careful charting of doses and effects by the patient. Experienced cannabis health care providers who have years of experience treating complex patients may recommend more aggressive or specific starting regimens. However, patients and providers who are relatively new to cannabis medicine will find that these recommendations are based on the desire to avoid side effects and the intent to relieve symptoms without impairment.

Another important consideration for patients using ingested cannabis product is the time lapse between ingestion and full effect. Orally ingested products may take one to three hours to have full effect, and those effects may last six to eight hours. Therefore, I strongly recommend *not* to re-dose oral cannabis products for at least three to four hours. Beware delayed cumulative action of oral cannabis as ingesting too much can have prolonged unpleasant side effects.

Due to the prolonged action of oral cannabis, usually there is no therapeutic benefit from increasing oral cannabis dosing beyond every four- to six-hour frequency, which corresponds to four times daily use as a maximum. In fact, usually two times daily (BID) to three times daily (TID) dosing is sufficient for the majority of patients. If symptoms persist despite four times daily (QID) dosing, then either increase dose, change product, or consider using a rapid onset inhalation product for "breakthrough" symptom relief. Patients should keep a journal and document dose, frequency, results of treatment, and side effects.

Dosing for Inhalation

Most medical cannabis consumers are currently choosing to use oral ingestion, which is not surprising since most conventional medicines are also swallowed by mouth. Inhalation is falling out of favour, particularly since it's associated with smoking, which is not recommended for medical use. However, the inhalational route of consumption is common and beneficial in some areas of conventional medicine. Inhalational consumption methods for medications used to treat asthma and other respiratory conditions include nebulizers, puffers, and inhalers. Inhalation also has medical benefits in some situations with cannabis, and while future options for inhaling cannabis will likely include nebulizers and metered dose inhalers, currently vaporizing is available and is much safer than traditional smoking. Experienced cannabis educators, found at many cannabis clinics, can teach patients how to use inhaled cannabis by vaporizer effectively.

Inhaled cannabis has a faster onset, shorter duration, and more intense effect than orally ingested cannabis. Onset is typically in one to ten minutes and effects typically last for one to three hours. Therefore, I recommend inhalation for patients with severe symptoms who require rapid onset of effect. Health Canada recommends that to convert an oral dose to an estimated inhaled dose, divide the oral dose by 2.5.[261] While it's not medically necessary to follow this conversion precisely, it does emphasize that a dose of inhaled cannabis has a potentially much stronger effect than a dose of oral cannabis. Because of this more intense and powerful effect, inhaled medical cannabis should be used only with caution and under the advice of a health care provider. In general, it should not be used in safety-sensitive workplace situations or when driving. For patients new to inhaled cannabis, starting low and going slow is very important as is using the medicine carefully at home until effects, and side effects, are determined.

To inhale cannabis medicine, I recommend vaporizing rather than smoking since, when vaporized, cannabinoids are boiled into vapour rather than combusted into smoke, producing significantly less toxic by-product. Start with one to two puffs (gentle mid-inhalation as deep, aggressive inhalation can produce unpleasant coughing). Typically, each inhalation will give a similar dose to standard edible but the exact dose depends on many factors, including cannabis strength and vaporizer temperature. Again, because inhaled cannabis typically has a faster onset, shorter duration, and more intense effect than ingested cannabis, a careful and cautious approach to dosing is indicated. Wait at least ten to twenty minutes before taking additional doses of inhaled cannabis and remember that some cannabis strains have a "creeper effect" with delayed full onset. Effects of inhaled cannabis typically last from one to three hours. Since the duration of action is shorter than for edible products, re-dosing can occur more often and patients may find themselves needing to repeat use every two to three hours. This frequency can make keeping control of symptoms at work difficult and is a reason many patients use background oral medicine for its prolonged effects. They may then use inhaled cannabis only occasionally when symptoms flare or breakthrough despite oral medicine use.

Traditional smoking via pipe, bong, or joint is not recommended for health reasons, since inhalation of any type of smoke into the lungs has significant potential health risks. However, some patients get advice from friends or experienced cannabis users who believe that the benefits of the whole plant effect can be best achieved with traditional smoking delivery. There is no good scientific proof of the validity of this concept, but some experienced traditional cannabis users continue to report better relief when using whole plant smoke inhalation. Those who choose to use medical cannabis by smoking, despite advice against this, can typically expect to use 0.25 g to 0.5 g of dry herb per joint or pipe/bong bowl. With this method, the initial dose is one to two mid-inhalation puffs from the joint, pipe, or bong. As with vaporizing, wait at least ten to twenty minutes to determine the full effect before taking additional doses.

When ordering product for inhalation delivery, the grams per day applies to dried flower, which is sold by weight in grams. Therefore, no conversion is needed. For a patient requiring oil product for background use as well as dried flower for inhalational breakthrough symptom relief, a health care provider needs to authorize enough grams per day dried cannabis equivalent for ordering oils as well as additional quantity to allow ordering the required dry flower.

Adjusting Dosage

The effects of cannabis medicine depend on many factors, including the dose, the types of cannabinoids, the delivery method, and the individual responses of the patient. Just like any medicine, some patients will find that cannabis medicine is just not effective or can't be tolerated. Typically, the effects of inhaled cannabis are noticed within seconds or minutes, whereas the effects of oral cannabis medicine may not be noticed for more than an hour. As cannabis medicine is usually started at extremely low doses (start low and go slow), it's likely that patients won't notice anything dramatic at all. With a careful and slow therapeutic trial, it may take days or weeks to notice any clear benefit or effect. Unlike opiates, which can be like a sledgehammer in terms of effects (and side effects), carefully taken cannabis medicine may be much more subtle. The improvement may be slow and gentle, but remember that the goal is relief of symptoms without side effects. The costs of this approach are that it requires more patient and provider engagement and that it takes effort and time. The benefits are that patients are using a safe natural medicine that can relieve multiple symptoms and may help get them off other more harmful pharmaceuticals.

Once patients obtain a medical cannabis authorization and receive products from a safe, regulated LP source, the dosing and titration process begins. Patients will help determine effective dosing through a slow and methodical process that will include documentation and journalling. Patients should keep a detailed record of what cannabis medicines they take, how and when they take them, and in what doses. It's also critical for patients to document what positive effects and side effects occur. Setting a target or a goal in terms of symptom relief is also helpful. As an example, a patient's goal could be a 50 percent reduction in arthritic knee pain without any side effects. The patient could then document that a certain dose caused minimal reduction in pain with no side effects, a higher dose caused moderate reduction in pain with no side effects, and the highest dose caused almost complete elimination of pain but with enough dizziness that walking was difficult. In that trial, a moderate reduction of pain with no side effects is likely the optimal outcome. If satisfied, the patient could then continue with the optimal regimen. If the trial is unsuccessful in meeting the treatment goals, a new cannabis product with a different cannabinoid profile could be tried.

As mentioned above, some patients and health care providers will enjoy this process, and others won't. While the lack of strict dosing recommendations may be frustrating for some patients and providers, self-directed adjustment does give significant control and flexibility for patients, allowing them active participation in the process of improving their own well-being.

Let's take a closer look at how a patient would begin cannabis treatment using the start-low, go-slow approach. With this approach, patients will start on a minimal dose that has almost zero likelihood of side effects. The dose can then be slowly increased (titrated) over days or weeks, and patients will document results in their treatment journal. These results are then reviewed in a follow-up appointment with the health care provider, and adjustments are made until the patient achieves an optimal dosing schedule.

The lowest possible dose of medical cannabis currently available would be one or two drops of standard cannabis oil or one puff of inhaled cannabis. It's not really feasible to take less than one drop of liquid medicine or less than one puff of inhaled medicine. Those minimal doses correlate to approximately 2.5 mg of active cannabinoid in most available oils and most inhaled medical cannabis products. An initial starting dose that low has essentially zero risk of serious negative side effects and usually needs to be slowly increased to obtain the desired relief of symptoms. If a patient experiences any undesirable side effects, the current dose and/or frequency of use should be decreased. If a dose and frequency that helps to improve symptoms without bothersome side effects can't be found, then another formulation of cannabis medicine with a different THC:CBD ratio should be considered. In the case of inhaled dried flower product, the composition of other cannabis chemical compounds sometimes also determines the effects for the individual patient. Since we are lacking any validated science-based guidelines to make recommendations on these other cannabis chemicals, this discussion is limited to THC and CBD. Remember that most of the potential negative side effects of cannabis are the result of only one cannabinoid, THC. Decreasing the THC dose, or increasing the ratio of CBD, which counters THC side effects, is often all that is required.

As already mentioned, with the start-low, go-slow approach, a patient may initially experience no effects at all, either positive or negative. This is fine and not uncommon when starting with such a minimal dose of cannabis. It's an incredibly safe approach, and really the only downside is the extra time it will take to titrate upward to an effective dose. There are a number of important reasons for emphasizing the principle of starting slowly with a very small dose. First, bothersome side effects are extremely rare at low doses whereas beneficial effects are quite common. Second, cannabis medicine can occasionally produce a paradoxical effect at high doses. This means that while low-dose cannabis medicine may relieve bothersome symptoms, high-dose cannabis may actually worsen those symptoms. This opposite effect with high-dose cannabis is especially true with high-THC products that are more commonly used as recreational agents. To avoid the risk of experiencing this paradoxical effect, always start low and go slow. Finally, starting with a low dose is the safest approach given that we lack data to guide dosing recommendations. Cannabis is remarkably safe, and initiating therapy with the start-low, go-slow approach makes it even safer.

Even for patients who are veteran recreational cannabis consumers, the same careful dosing schedule should apply. As these patients begin to intentionally use pharmaceutical-grade cannabis for medical purposes, they should adjust recreational expectations and habits and seek a moderate dose with maximum therapeutic benefit. Recreational cannabis is typically used to maximize psychoactive and euphoric side effects. Medical cannabis is used to relieve symptoms with as little impairment as possible. Relief of symptoms without impairment or harm is the key goal of medical cannabis therapy.

In summary, the take-home message is that cannabis medicine doesn't have to be complicated for patients or providers but does require a careful and methodical approach to maximize potential benefit of therapy. It's incredibly safe and the risk of harms at very low doses is negligible. Cannabis medicine is often effective at doses far lower than those required to cause side effects. Therefore, the start-low, go-slow recommendation helps patients find the dose of cannabis medicine that works for them while hopefully avoiding unpleasant side effects. Until future research trials are able to define more specific dosing guidelines, cannabis therapy will remain highly individualized and slow titration will often be required to find the most effective dose.

PART IV
USING MEDICAL CANNABIS

Cannabis medicine is not new, but its re-emergence into a scientifically and technologically sophisticated world is. The result is that we are witnessing a rapid and almost explosive release of pent-up demand, cannabis-related research, and sophisticated new products and devices developed specifically for the medical market. Consequently, a more in-depth discussion of how we can use medical cannabis in Canada today, and where we may be going in the future, is worthwhile.

CHAPTER 10

OBTAINING MEDICAL CANNABIS

Now that cannabis is legal for both recreational and medical purposes, Canadians have a number of options for obtaining cannabis products. While black market street cannabis has always been available, it will remain as unknown product with undetermined source, content, and contaminants. The only source of safe, legal, regulated cannabis for purchase in Canada remains the LPs, the number and diversity of which are growing.

Smaller LPs may opt to specialize in their product lines and may not choose to participate in both the recreational and medical markets. Most of the large Canadian producers will likely begin to offer both product lines, although some larger producers will likely produce cannabis wholesale to be sold only to other LPs for marketing and distribution.

The emphasis on more detailed and refined medical cannabis research will inevitably lead to development and production of specific cannabinoid blends, some of which may ultimately be produced synthetically in the laboratory. These products will likely receive DINs and be available to patients by prescription through licensed pharmacies. Many of these possibilities remain speculative, and the Canadian medical cannabis patient will continue obtaining medical cannabis by either purchasing from an LP, growing it themselves, or designating an authorized grower.

LICENSED PRODUCERS

Canadian LPs are currently the only regulated producers, and usually also distributors, of legal medical cannabis under the ACMPR regulations and the Cannabis Act. Some patients may wonder what the difference is between an LP and a dispensary. Prior to recreational legalization, all dispensaries were illegal operations. After recreational legalization, the intent is for regulated dispensaries to be locations for on-site sale of recreational products from one or more LPs. In some provinces and municipalities, an LP will be permitted to have an on-site dispensary. This would be a little like a retail store selling wine on the premises of a vineyard.

The requirement to purchase from one of these regulated LPs may seem onerous to some Canadians, particularly if they were used to purchasing from one of the many illegal dispensaries. However, before judging the LP system, patients should consider a number of significant advantages to purchasing from regulated sources. Most important is that the system provides access to safe, regulated, uncontaminated, medical-grade product. The same is not true of the black market or illegal dispensaries where studies have shown that up to 80 percent of products contain some form of contamination, including pesticides, insecticides, fungi, mould, and other drugs. Additionally, medical products from LPs are increasingly labelled with detailed information stating amount and type of cannabinoids present, unlike illegal cannabis, which is often of unknown composition and quality.

LPs produce cannabis under stringent guidelines and regulations, including Good Production Practices, and many are also introducing the more stringent Good Manufacturing Practices. These regulations are the same ones under which the food and pharmaceutical industries operate. The goal of these practices is to ensure that Canadian patients access safe, quality-controlled medical product that is free of both pesticides and other potentially harmful contaminants. From a harm-reduction standpoint alone, using medical grade products from regulated LPs is much safer than self-medicating with street product.

By licensing and regulating corporations to legally produce cannabis in Canada and subjecting them to strict safety checks and quality controls, Health Canada has established the parameters for a largely unprecedented industry and has positioned Canadian LPs at the leading edge of cannabis research and development worldwide. The cannabis supplied by Canada's own LPs is among the best available, and demand for these cannabis products extends to countries across the planet. The large Canadian LPs are currently the world's leading cannabis companies in terms of research, production, export agreements, and stock value.

Choosing a Licensed Producer

When accessing medical cannabis by purchasing product directly from one of Health Canada's LPs, Canadians can choose from well over one hundred companies, though only about half this number are actively producing and distributing products. The growing number of LPs allows each company to concentrate on offering specific and specialized products, often competing to offer medical patients the best oils or whole plant strains for the lowest price. There are so many LPs that choosing among them can be a difficult decision. Current regulations allow patients to split their grams-per-day authorization among a number of LPs, but patients must still limit their choices significantly among all LPs that are available. Whether an LP is a good fit for an individual patient depends on what factors are important for that patient. Those factors may include customer service, price point, product type, shipping efficiency and costs, availability of compassionate pricing, and availability of educational information. It's also common for patients to choose an LP based on their geographical location as many people prefer a local LP that produces product in the town or province where they live.

Product availability is often a major factor influencing patient LP choice. Not all LPs offer ingestible oils or gelcaps, and many smaller LPs only offer a selection of dried cannabis flower. Other LPs may offer fairly generic products but pride themselves on pricing, processing registration efficiently, and offering same-day shipping. Ultimately, the factors that appeal to each patient will help to determine which LP they choose. Sometimes the choice comes down to ordering from a producer that is in the same town or region, as local pride often influences purchase decisions. As the industry matures and new research shows benefit of different cannabinoid preparations, the LP market will likely continue to increase product specialization. Product offerings will therefore likely be a major future factor in LP choice. For instance, if a particular LP has a patented blend shown to help MS patients, most of those patients will choose to make their purchases there.

When it comes to choosing an LP, even extensive personal research may be insufficient for some patients to choose one specific company among all the others. This need to choose a producer of their medicine can be frustrating for some patients, as they are not asked to choose which company they want to purchase their other conventional medicines from. Usually, we just take prescriptions for medications to the pharmacy and pick up the medicine when it's ready. Just as patients rely on their local pharmacy to choose quality sources of prescription medicines, patients may depend on the guidance of cannabis industry experts for LP choice.

Currently, most busy conventional health care providers do not have all the individual LP information or the extra time to sort this information out. Many of them choose to refer their patients to cannabis clinics for this reason. That is why experienced medical cannabis clinics will have an education team on site, including experts in LP information, prepared to discuss this decision with the patient as soon as they finish their appointment with a dedicated cannabis physician. The ability to provide on-site education and LP guidance is one of the reasons so many patients are being referred by their health care providers to legitimate specialty cannabis clinics. Speaking with a dedicated cannabis clinic educator is often a vital step in completing a cannabis clinic appointment and becoming a medical cannabis patient. Not only will these educators help patients to find an appropriate LP that meets their needs, but they will also guide patients through the registration process so the medical document can be sent to the LP.

Legitimate medical cannabis clinics should be unbiased and have a mandate to help patients choose an LP in an agnostic manner. Ideally, their recommendations should be supported by knowledgeable experts and up-to-date information on all LP offerings. If a particular clinic is unable to offer comprehensive information on multiple producers, it may be directing patients toward a particular LP with which it partners. Patients should be cautious of this bias since when it comes to selling medically specific products to medical patients, any exclusive relationships between medical clinics and individual LPs or dispensaries is prohibited.

Even with expert guidance, evaluating LPs is difficult because the industry is still maturing and evolving. The landscape that exists today will likely be very different than the one that exists even a year from now. By the time this book is printed, it's likely that some of the information may already be out of date. However, now that Health Canada has declared that the ACMPR regulations will be kept in place for at least five years, the medical market should have some stability. The effect of recreational cannabis legalization is undoubtedly going to change the medical LP market, but possibly not in ways that were initially predicted. Some in the industry assumed that recreational legalization would depress the medical market, but instead the opposite appears to be happening. With rising demand for medical cannabis, LPs are starting to compete for patients. More LPs are offering compassionate pricing, which is reduced pricing for legitimate medical patients who can't afford medication purchase. We have also seen an increase in free shipping on medical products and introduction of new medical product offerings. Already, many LPs are announcing that they will cover the tax on medical products for legitimate medical patients with official medical authorization.

Registering with a Licensed Producer

All LPs have a similar registration process to authorize patient accounts. This process has two main components. The first is completion of the online registration form, found on the LP website. The second is receipt of a signed medical document from the authorizing health care provider. Many LPs have adopted a registration system that uses secure and compliant software programs. Using these platforms, LPs are able to auto-populate the information on a patient's medical document directly into the registration form. The patient's account is then securely authorized as soon as the medical document is sent.

This authorization usually requires that both the health care provider's office where the medical document is generated and the LP are using the same compliant software. Without this software link, the process of completing and sending a medical cannabis document and getting a patient registered with an LP can be time consuming and inefficient for both the provider and patient. While more providers are now getting compliant medical cannabis software in their offices, the potential difficulties of medical document generation and patient LP registration continue to be a major reason that many non-cannabis providers refer their patients to specialty cannabis clinics. The reality is that most Canadian health care providers don't have the time, expertise, or software integration required to send the medical cannabis documents to LPs in a secure and efficient manner.

At the more experienced cannabis clinics, this entire procedure will be coordinated by an education team that will summarize relevant LP information, guide patients to the one that precisely fits their needs, help with the registration process, and ensure that the medical document is sent securely and immediately to the correct LP.

Changing and Choosing Multiple Licensed Producers

An obvious question with the initial ACMPR was what happened if patients wanted to switch LPs. They may have initially chosen an LP only to discover that they didn't like the product, they had trouble with customer service, or the LP suddenly increased prices. Fortunately, the revised regulations under the Cannabis Act make LP changes easier for the patient. The new regulations do not bind patients to any LPs that they initially choose. Under the new Cannabis Act, patients have the right to request an active medical document back from their current LP so that they can sign up with a new one. They also have the right to request transfer of the medical document from one LP to another. Additionally, as long as patients are working with a health care provider's office that has a compliant way to send medical documents to LPs, it's fairly easy to send part of their grams-per-day authorization to one LP for oils and to a different LP for another product.

It's possible, although somewhat challenging, for patients to make these changes on their own, and until cannabis medicine becomes better integrated with conventional medicine, it's often easier for both patients and providers to work with legitimate cannabis clinics. Every medical clinic will have different policies and procedures concerning this action, and some will likely be more accommodating than others. How flexible a medical clinic will be in facilitating a change of LP registration usually depends on their size and experience.

Ordering Cannabis Medicine

Once registered with an LP, patients can proceed with ordering their cannabis medicine, which will be delivered to their home address by courier or postal service within a matter of days. Under previous ACMPR rules, patients were able to order only thirty days' worth of cannabis medicine at a time, up to their maximum grams-per-day allotment. Due to shipping and delivery delays, this restriction sometimes resulted in patients running out of medicine. Under the Cannabis Act, these original ACMPR limitations have been removed, and patients are allowed to order more than a 30-day supply of medical cannabis at a time. To make it legal to store more than a one-month supply of medicine, the Cannabis Act does not limit personal storage quantities of cannabis at home.

In addition to ordering from LPs, under the Cannabis Act medical patients with an active medical document are also able to apply for a licence to grow their own medicine or designate someone to grow for them. In the future, patients will likely be able to purchase medical cannabis directly from a pharmacy, thus greatly reducing the delay between their medical appointment and the time they obtain their medication. Large pharmacy chains in Canada have applied for, and in some cases have already been granted, LP licences in order to meet this anticipated demand.

CHOOSING MEDICAL CANNABIS PRODUCTS

When choosing medical cannabis products, patients need to consider a number of factors, most importantly the recommendations of their health care providers. Such a variety of products is available that the choice can be overwhelming, and the greatest likelihood of achieving relief of symptoms without side effects will be through a careful process that requires active patient and provider engagement. The primary decisions to be made include whether the patient will use dry flower for inhalation or cannabis oils for ingestion, whether they prefer an approach based on ratios of the primary cannabinoids, CBD and THC, or if they want to consider the potential therapeutic benefits of other cannabis compounds, including terpenes, for which there is currently less scientific support.

Oils versus Flowers

Under the original ACMPR, only two main product types were available from Canadian LPs: dried cannabis flower and cannabis extracts in ingestible oils, and at the time of this writing those are still all that are currently available. However, already LPs are being creative and are using the allowed products to create more delivery options. One LP offers an oil product as a sublingual spray, while another offers a base topical cream that can be mixed with available oils to make topical medicine. This limited product selection will change soon as the new Cannabis Act promises access to a wider range of medical products. In addition to the currently available products, a number of LPs are working on a variety of premixed topical cannabis medicines, tablet formulations, metered dose inhalers, and transdermal patches.

Because most conventional medications are taken by mouth, most medical cannabis patients prefer to start taking their cannabis medicine this way. Therefore, edible oils used in either droppers or gelcaps are currently the most popular medical cannabis products. In addition to the fact that patients tend to prefer oral medications, choosing and shopping for ingestible oils and gelcaps is usually much simpler than choosing dried flower. Most LPs have a limited number of oil extracts available, differentiated primarily by cannabinoid profile. The relative simplicity of this limited range of oils and the straightforward dosing schedule afforded by ingestible oils (measured in millilitres) are attractive factors for new cannabis patients and often also for providers.

In contrast, when choosing dried cannabis flower for medical purposes, patients traditionally have had to choose among a huge number of different strains, often with confusing names and lists of unfamiliar-sounding chemicals. Much of this diversity came from the fact that patients were previously self-medicating with recreational cannabis varietals that often kept their original names and descriptions. Recreational legalization has actually helped this situation since many LPs are now producing a more limited line of dried flower products for the medical patient, with product labelling more clearly stating cannabinoid profiles, terpene profiles, and anticipated medical uses and effects. While the extensive variety of available dried cannabis flower can still be overwhelming, experienced cannabis consumers accustomed to inhaling cannabis or those interested in a wider variety of products may still prefer to purchase dried flower.

Cannabinoid Profile

The cannabinoid profile is likely the most important consideration when choosing a medical cannabis product, and it's ultimately the factor that will determine the product's beneficial effects and potential side effects. Although the cannabis plant contains dozens of unique cannabinoid compounds and hundreds of additional plant chemicals, it's the two primary compounds, THC and CBD, that result in most of its proven beneficial effects.

Choosing a medical cannabis oil tends to be a fairly simple process. The vast majority of oils available from Canadian LPs can be divided into three primary categories: THC predominant, CBD predominant, and balanced THC and CBD. Oil products usually express THC and CBD as a milligram dose per millilitre of oil (for example, THC 5 mg/mL). Since most cannabis side effects are THC related, many patients choose to start with CBD-predominant oil. These oils are called "CBD predominant" rather than "CBD pure" since they are made with whole plant extracts that always have at least a tiny component of THC. While this reality may be a problem for patients working in jobs with a zero-THC policy, from a medical perspective it may be beneficial as evidence suggests that at least some THC is required for CBD to work optimally. However, this concept still needs to be validated with good research data. In cases where CBD-predominant oil doesn't help, the next choice is usually a balanced THC–CBD product. THC-predominant preparations are usually limited to use in situations where patients have achieved less benefit with lower THC preparations or in conditions where data specifically points to benefit of THC, as discussed in more detail in Part III.

Similar considerations regarding cannabinoid profile apply when choosing among strains of dried flower. While online reviews and experience of other medical patients with regard to particular strains (which I discuss later in this section) may be useful, the primary decision often comes down to choosing a relative strength of THC, usually expressed in dried flower by percentage of THC by weight. While the same decision now applies to percentage of CBD, until recently most traditionally available recreational strains were very low in CBD (less than 1 percent) and the percentage of CBD was not usually reported. With high-CBD strains becoming increasingly available on the market, product labelling is starting to accommodate these new consumer choices. Dried recreational cannabis often has a THC content of 20 to 25 percent or higher. While this much THC is likely to produce an effective and desirable euphoriant experience for the recreational user, most medical patients will find cannabis flower of this potency much stronger than they need and much more likely to produce side effects. Dried flower medical products usually have reduced THC side effects with a THC content of 15 percent or less.

Additionally, while most recreational cannabis has less than 1 percent CBD, by combining plant genetics into hybrid plants, growers have now developed cannabis strains that produce balanced CBD and THC profiles. Since CBD helps combat THC side effects, these strains can be particularly helpful to medical patients. Welcome news to medical patients is that an increasing number of CBD-predominant strains are becoming available. These strains may be as high as 20 percent CBD and as low as 0.5 percent THC, providing relief of inflammation, anxiety, and other CBD-related medical conditions with almost no risk of psychoactivity or impairment. As the medical cannabis industry progresses, medical cannabis patients will have access to a much broader range of medical cannabis formulations and devices. In this sense, while medical cannabis is ancient, advanced medical delivery systems and medically specific formulations are just beginning.

It's important to understand the potential limits of the content information provided by LPs. Stated THC and CBD percentages on dried cannabis products have historically tended to be rough estimates and were often not totally accurate. The situation is improving with regulations now requiring increased testing and accurate labelling of available products. The percentage of THC or CBD indicated in a given dried product should ideally be presented in a range as the percentage of cannabinoids actually present is affected by the moisture content and overall weight. The more moisture present in the product, the more it will weigh and the lower the relative THC percentage will be. Some labs test completely dried product to eliminate the effects of moisture on the percentage calculations, but most don't. The actual product sold will typically have more moisture and, therefore, a slightly lower relative THC or CBD content than the sample tested. Oil-based extracts should theoretically be easier to test and analyze due to elimination of the water moisture variable. However, cannabis analytic testing is a relatively new requirement, and as yet there are very few universally accepted standards for cannabis analytics. Consequently, it's still quite possible that variations in results will occur from one lab to another, even when testing identical product. This inconsistency should improve with time as testing regulations and laboratory cannabis protocols become more accepted and standardized.

Another issue with content information is that a given batch of cannabis may have a great deal of variation from plant to plant and flower to flower. Where the tested sample was obtained influences the test results and may influence whether the sample was representative or not. For example, if a producer holds 5 g from each lot to confirm potency levels but makes 50,000 g batches, it's not hard to imagine how the reading can change based on which 5 g were sent to the lab. Therefore, knowing exact percentages of cannabinoids in dried flower remains a challenge in cannabis medicine, but it's likely not that important to the consumer since finding the best product and most effective dosing usually requires adjustment and experimentation anyway. Labelling dried cannabis product with a range of percentages is probably more accurate and useful and is already being practised by some LPs.

Terpene Profile

As previously discussed, terpenes, or plant essential oils, are an exciting yet poorly understood aspect of cannabis medicine. Many cannabis scientists believe that these compounds have their own therapeutic effects and may also help to increase the efficacy of cannabis medicine overall. This concept has not been well validated, however, and most research on cannabis as medicine has concentrated on the two primary cannabinoids, THC and CBD. While the terpenes indeed may contribute to the effectiveness of medical cannabis, little specific research currently supports their contribution to an added therapeutic effect.

Recreational users, however, report significantly different effects depending on the terpene profile of the strain in question. Cannabis strains high in the terpene myrcene are known to be sedating and relaxing, whereas strains high in the terpene limonene tend to be more uplifting and mood enhancing. The terpene pinene is a known bronchodilator, and high pinene strains have been anecdotally reported as beneficial in asthmatics. As research data emerge, more and more producers are including proprietary terpenoid blends to try and take advantage of the reported therapeutic properties of these chemicals. Many LPs have started to list primary terpenes and reported benefits on their dried flower ordering charts, and some have started to list terpene profiles in their oil products as well.

Strains

In addition to cannabinoid and terpene profiles, patients will find a range of available strains when choosing medical cannabis products. You'll remember from Part II that cannabis strains usually come from one of two main accepted varietals, sativa and indica, or a hybrid of both. Despite the debate about the relevance of the differentiation and the fact that the vast majority of modern cannabis strains are hybrids, most cannabis products are still marketed and sold as either sativa or indica. While it's popular to attribute a range of typical effects to either sativa, indica, or hybrid strains, the reliable indicators of the strain's effect will be in its tested THC and CBD content and, to a lesser extent, the terpene profile. As discussed in the previous section, LPs will also indicate a percentage of both THC and CBD for each strain they offer, and this ratio may ultimately be the more important consideration for the medical patient.

A tremendous amount of information regarding the myriad of traditionally available cannabis strains is available online. This information typically includes advice on which strains are best for which conditions and what kind of experience a patient can expect from each one. Much of this information is not based on scientifically rigorous data, has very little to substantiate its claims besides anecdotal evidence, and should be used with caution. Underlying the reality that the abundant online strain information is often dubious are a number of facts. First, there are no universally agreed-upon principles for naming cannabis strains, and one grower's Purple Kush may be a totally different plant strain with very different chemical profile than another grower's. Second, studies have shown that even genetically identical plants may produce different profiles of medical cannabis compounds depending on the environmental growing conditions. This environmental variation is similar to how winemakers can produce very different wines using the same grapes grown in different soil conditions.

Finally, validated cannabis testing and analytics are currently inconsistent, particularly those outside the LP system. A given dried flower product may have very different testing results from one lab to another. Despite these inconsistencies, the information that each LP provides about its specific products is likely of reasonable quality since most LP products require both internal and external validated testing of components. Therefore, although strain information provided by LPs might not be perfect, it's typically better than most general online reviews of a particular named strain. In time, the industry may mature enough to allow universal classification and compositional analysis, but that is likely many years away. In the meantime, cannabis medicines are likely to be increasingly studied and sold as specific known quantities of individual cannabis chemicals rather than as plant strains.

Controlling Side Effects

One of the most common assumptions about medical cannabis is that cannabis will always intoxicate its users or make them "high." The concept was supported in earlier cannabis studies that looked at side effects of cannabis in patients who were self-medicating with recreational product. This belief that a person has to get high to achieve symptom relief is a reason that many people are still against cannabis medicine. Even a cursory look at the modern medical cannabis literature will tell you that this common belief is not true. Not all cannabis products are intoxicating, and the symptom relief provided by cannabis does not necessarily extend from the dissociative high that it can produce. The goal of all medical therapy, including cannabis therapy, is relief of symptoms without side effects or impairment.

For most medical cannabis consumers, the prospect of cannabis intoxication is both unpleasant and inconvenient. It represents an unwanted side effect of a medication they hope to use without impairment during the day, while at work, to control pain or regulate other symptoms. Whether or not medical cannabis will cause intoxication or impairment depends in large part on its full chemical profile, the dose used, and whether it has a high percentage of THC or is balanced with CBD to mitigate the THC effects. It also depends on the sensitivity of the individual patient to the plant chemicals.

The remarkable success stories of pediatric patients achieving return of function after remission of disabling drug-resistant epilepsy by using high-CBD, low-THC cannabis show that symptom relief without functional impairment is not only optimal but actually possible. Even THC, which definitely can cause intoxication and impairment, often produces relief of symptoms at doses far lower than those required to get a recreational high. Canadian patients in increasing numbers are discovering that slowly titrating doses of medical cannabis products usually allows relief of symptoms while controlling and avoiding side effects.

GROWING YOUR OWN CANNABIS

With the ACMPR grow-at-home program, cannabis patients who want complete control over their medicine production can buy seeds or cloned plants from LPs. Often, this method will produce a larger and more immediately accessible stock of medicine, while ensuring that patients are getting exactly the products they desire. The ACMPR also permits patients to nominate a designated grower, allowing them to outsource the labour while retaining their own private stock of home-grown cannabis. Below, I review the details of these regulations and how the revisions of the Cannabis Act have affected medical cannabis patients.

Grow-at-Home Provisions

The revised ACMPR rules still allow for patients to apply for permission to grow cannabis for medical purposes at home. Under the new Cannabis Act, all Canadians of legal age are also allowed to grow up to four plants for recreational purposes, provided the seeds or plants come from approved sources. Given this provision, it may seem strange that Health Canada still requires an authorized medical document to grow cannabis for medical purposes. Medical cannabis patients may therefore wonder if the ACMPR program is still relevant. Because it allows patients to grow more cannabis than the recreational laws, it indeed still is. For patients with large cannabis needs, the provisions of the recreational Cannabis Act would be insufficient as these patients would need to grow more than the allotted four plants at a time to meet the higher grams-per-day allotment on their medical documents. Under the ACMPR program, patients can obtain a registration certificate from Health Canada that allows them to possess more cannabis in public than would otherwise be allowed for recreational consumers. Because medical cannabis patients can legally grow and possess significantly more cannabis than recreational users, the ACMPR's grow-at-home program may actually see more traffic since passage of the Cannabis Act rather than less.

The number of plants a patient can grow through the current ACMPR's grow-at-home program depends on the grams-per-day authorization on the medical document, where the patient chooses to grow the plants (indoors, outdoors, or both), and the typical number of growth cycles expected each year under those conditions. Health Canada's calculations assume that plants grown indoors will produce fewer grams of flower than plants grown outdoors and that indoor growing allows for more growth cycles than outdoor growing. These assumptions affect the calculations for number of plants patients can grow under their grams-per-day medical document authorization. The calculations used to determine the number of plants a patient can grow are provided in the table below for easy reference.

Table 1: ACMPR grow-at-home allowances for indoor and outdoor medical cannabis plants

Growing conditions	Allowed number of plants, multiplied by the daily grams authorized	
	Indoor plants	Outdoor plants
Indoors only	5	0
Outdoors only	0	2
Both indoors and outdoors	4	1

If growing only indoors, patients are allowed to grow five times the number of plants as daily grams authorized. If growing only outdoors, patients are allowed to grow two times the number of plants as daily grams authorized. Patients planning to grow both indoors and outdoors may grow four times the number of *indoor* plants and the same number of *outdoor* plants as daily grams authorized. For example, if prescribed 5 g/day, a patient could grow twenty-five indoor plants only, ten outdoor plants only, or twenty indoor plants and five outdoor plants. The number of plants allowed includes those of any size or stage, from new starter clones to fully mature flowering plants. Simply put, any seed that has germinated counts under the plant allotment until it's harvested. Previously, the grow-at-home calculations specified a corresponding allowed home storage limit. Since the new Cannabis Act has removed all home storage limits for canna-bis, these storage limit numbers are now irrelevant. Given the caveat that home storage limits no longer apply, Health Canada provides an online calculator that computes the allowed number of plants. You can find a link to this calculator in the Resources section.

Application Process

The first step for patients who want to grow their own cannabis for medical purposes is applying to Health Canada for a registration certificate for personal or designated production. The application is available online as a fillable PDF and must be accompanied by the patient's original medical document. The application includes ques-tions about the patient's residence, their intended site of cannabis production, and whether cannabis will be stored at home or at the production site. Though properly completed applications will general-ly be accepted by Health Canada, the application itself can be difficult to navigate and its approval can take a long time. Since the grow-at-home program remains an important option for many patients, I've included in-depth instructions for completing the application in the Resources section at the end of the book.

The grow-at-home process under the original ACMPR made it difficult for some patients to successfully obtain a certificate from Health Canada. The application form is eleven pages long and be-comes potentially even more complex if a patient decides to specify a designated grower other than themselves. Additionally, the original medical document needs to be attached to the application form. As discussed earlier, prior to the new Cannabis Act patients rarely had easy access to their original documents. While patients always had a right to obtain a copy of their original medical document if requested, the Cannabis Act now states that they can get the original back from an LP. Therefore, it should be possible for a patient to complete the grow-at-home registration process on their own. For some patients, however, completion of the grow-at-home document is a complicated enough process that they choose to enlist the help of their medical cannabis clinic to effectively complete the application process. Some cannabis clinics have experienced staff members who are able to verify all relevant information, oversee the process, and attach the medical document.

Often, a complete and correct application is only the first step in a potentially slow process. Since inception of the grow-at-home program, Health Canada has become intermittently bogged down and the response time to grow-at-home applications and renewals has been difficult to predict. Health Canada has stated their average processing times for these applications is six to ten weeks. In reality, both first-time applications and renewals have occasionally taken more than six months to process.

So far, Health Canada has not been able to find a way to expedite or simplify this process, although it's possible that allowing recreational consumers to grow up to four plants without registration may help reduce backlog. Until the approval process speeds up, patients who wish to grow their own cannabis medicine should plan to submit their applications as soon as possible after receiving their medical documents to ensure their prescriptions don't expire before the approval process is complete. For the same reasons, patients wishing to renew their applications need to do so in a timely manner. Coordinating applications and renewals within the limited time windows has proved difficult for some patients in the past.

CHAPTER 11

CONSUMPTION AND OTHER DELIVERY METHODS

Before patients can start using cannabis, they need to choose the consumption or delivery method they will use. While this may seem obvious, the decision is something many new cannabis consumers don't consider. Taking cannabis medicine is quite different from most prescription medicines for which the prescribing health care provider makes these decisions. Currently, Canadian health care providers can make recommendations to patients but can't dictate the consumption method on the medical document. Even after discussing possible cannabis consumption methods with their health care providers, patients can still have difficulty choosing the most appropriate method.

Even experienced cannabis consumers often overlook a variety of consumption and delivery methods that could be beneficial. Getting the most from cannabis medicine may entail considering a variety of ways in which the medicine can be used. Additionally, it's important to understand that a tremendous amount of research is underway, looking into developing and perfecting more refined consumption and other delivery methods for medical cannabis. These methods include nebulizers, inhalers, buccal mucosal absorption strips, transdermal patches, tablets, topicals, sublingual sprays, and liquid preparations.

Let's begin by looking at four common methods used to consume or otherwise deliver medicine: inhalation, ingestion, topical

application, and suppository insertion. Within these categories, patients will find additional options, each with potential benefits and
drawbacks. However, with limited exceptions, at the time of this writing only products for inhalational and oral use are widely legally
available in Canada. Topical and suppository formats, along with other delivery options, are still being developed under the new Cannabis
Act. While a patient may be drawn to the potency and short-lived
effects of inhaling cannabis, that patient may also find benefit from
the prolonged effects of oral absorption or from directly applying cannabis to the site of inflammation with topicals.

Once patients begin to explore the relative benefits of different
consumption methods, they hopefully will find one or two that work
for them. As the medical cannabis industry matures, we'll likely
move toward consumption methods that are more in line with other
prescribed medicines, and in that case, the prescribing health care
provider will be more involved in recommending specific delivery
methods. In the meantime, patients have a lot of control over how
they take their cannabis medicine. Therefore, a more in-depth look at
consumption methods is worthwhile.

INHALATION DELIVERY METHODS

Inhalation delivery methods are often particularly useful for patients
suffering certain symptoms and ailments since cannabinoids have a
different onset and intensity of effect when inhaled than when ingested or applied in other manners. When inhaled, cannabis vapours or
gases enter through the lungs and are absorbed into the bloodstream,
resulting in a faster onset and briefer duration of effects when compared to oral ingestion. Since medicine goes straight from the lungs
to the heart and then directly to the brain, inhalation is usually also
associated with more pronounced and powerful effects. This effect is
one reason that inhaled medicines, such as rescue asthma inhalers or
nebulizers, are often used in urgent medical situations where rapid
onset and powerful effects are required. With cannabis medicine,
this brief but potent burst of cannabinoid uptake can help relieve
severe symptoms and can be a convenient delivery method for daytime use. This approach is often used for severe breakthrough pain in

users who are also on a background level of oral cannabis medicine. It can also be useful in patients with severe nausea and vomiting who need rapid onset of effects and also can't take medicines by mouth.

Most people associate cannabis consumption with inhalation delivery methods. While inhalation traditionally involved smoking a joint (a rolled cannabis cigarette) or inhaling smoke through a pipe or bong, smoking is never recommended for medical use. Inhaling smoke into the lungs can cause lung damage and harmful side effects. We know this, of course, from the abundance of studies performed on tobacco smoke. While studies show that cannabis smoke appears to be less harmful than cigarette smoke, inhaling any smoke into the lungs is potentially dangerous. In addition to potential personal harms, smoking cannabis produces second-hand smoke, which may distribute potential toxins and bothersome smoke to people in the immediate environment. It's also notorious for releasing a strong smell that can be unpleasant for bystanders. Therefore, medical cannabis providers recommend vaporizing over smoking if a patient decides on an inhalation delivery route.

Vaporizing is an important alternative to conventional smoking methods and should be seriously considered by all medical cannabis patients for its ability to neutralize the harmful effects of smoking. Vaporizing also uses the cannabis medicine more efficiently than smoking. Vaporizing boils, rather than combusts, the plant material, offering efficient extraction of the active plant compounds while eliminating over 90 percent of the toxins and carcinogens that are released by traditional combustion with smoking. Medical devices currently being developed, like nebulizers and metered-dose inhalers, will likely be safer and more accurate than either vaporizing or smoking and will likely be available for delivery of medical cannabis soon. Inhalational medical delivery devices are already common in the treatment of asthma and other breathing problems, so this concept is familiar to most patients.

Traditional Smoking Options
Although the bottom line from a medical perspective is that smoking is not recommended, smoking has been such a dominant part

of the cannabis culture for so long that ignoring it completely does not present an accurate picture. Before modern vaporizers and other inhalation devices were available, the simplest and easiest way to access the potential benefits of cannabis medicine was to light it on fire and inhale the smoke. Anyone familiar with cannabis culture has some awareness of the many ways to combust and smoke this plant. Rolled joints, artistic glass pipes, wooden pipes, single-use self-made pipes like an apple or a soda can with holes punched in them, hookahs, and water bongs continue to be popular among recreational cannabis users. Walking into a local pot shop often reveals a remarkable array of bongs and pipes, some of them elaborately ornamented.

Many of these traditional methods were once billed as having health benefits compared to direct joint smoking. The main argument was that they potentially introduced fewer toxins into the lungs. Using a water bong, for example, passes the smoke through water and reportedly filters out toxins. As there have been few scientific bong studies, the debate on this subject is ongoing with conflicting evidence to support both sides. While it's clear that the water is filtering some of the harmful polycyclic aromatic hydrocarbons and tar (a catch-all term for the toxic compounds in smoke), it may also be trapping some of those toxins in water droplets. Toxic compounds may then pass into the lungs with tiny water droplets, and dirty water could present a hazard. In the recreational community, regular users of water bongs are known to develop a nasty prolonged cough. Despite this potential hazard, the bong remains a favourite method among experienced recreational cannabis users. However, since they involve inhalation of smoke, bongs can't be endorsed by health professionals for medical use.

Other inhalation methods, such as hand pipes, have little to distinguish them as consumption methods besides their simplicity and sense of style and artistic expression. Smoking joints may have some appeal for those who have used cannabis to medicate their ailments for many years. It's easy, simple, and traditional. For those experienced with it, this method may allow cannabis consumers to regulate their dose precisely and afford all the comforts of simplicity and familiarity. Rolled joints are not subject to technical malfunction or battery drain. Joints are also inexpensive, which can allow some patients to have instant access to their medication rather than saving up for a potentially expensive vaporizer. Despite any potential benefits of these alternative smoking methods, however, smoking is still never recommended from a medical perspective.

Vaporizing

Vaporizing is a healthier choice for medical cannabis consumers who wish to experience the benefits of inhaled cannabis but not expose themselves to the known harmful effects of smoking. These benefits include a rapid onset of often powerful effects and the ability to adjust frequency of doses quickly and accurately.

A vaporizer heats cannabis to a specific set temperature, usually around 188 to 200°C, at which the plant's cannabinoids are extracted by boiling but potentially harmful toxins are not combusted or released. Vaporizers do not burn the cannabis and they do not produce smoke. They simply heat the cannabis to a temperature where the cannabinoids turn into vapour through boiling, and this vapour can be inhaled. Smoking, on the other hand, delivers cannabinoids and by-product toxins directly through high temperature (500 to 1000°C) burning/combustion. Vaporizing eliminates exposure to smoke-related carcinogens since smoke is not produced, allowing patients to take controlled, moderate puffs, usually with much less harsh feeling and coughing than smoking (though vaporizing high-THC extracts, which are not currently available from LPs, can produce bronchial irritation and coughing fits). Additionally, vaporizing mostly neutralizes the smell of cannabis, allowing patients to discreetly medicate. The by-product of a vaporizer is mist or vapour, not smoke. Despite this minimal impact, many businesses have a strict no smoking and no vaporizing policy.

Another benefit of vaporizing is more efficient use of potentially expensive cannabis medicine. Vaporizers use significantly less dried cannabis than do conventional smoke inhalation methods. Fire consumes cannabis quickly, whereas vaporizing slowly boils off the medicinal components. This efficient extraction allows patients to reduce waste and economize their supplies of medicine. Not only does vaporizing have the potential to increase the yield of cannabinoids that the patient receives, but it also leaves a non-burned by-product that looks like tobacco, typically brown with some yellowish-green hues. This leftover cannabis material still has a small amount of residual cannabinoid, and motivated patients can use it to make edibles, like cannabis butter, thereby providing another consumption option. Finally, the resin that builds up in a vaporizer, particularly with larger tabletop models, is also full of cannabinoids and can be re-vaporized for a more concentrated dose of medicine. Most cannabis users who switch from smoking to vaporizing notice they purchase much less cannabis, resulting in significant potential savings.

In Canada, at the time of this writing, medical cannabis patients will exclusively use dried cannabis flower in vaporizers. However, with the expanding range of both legal and illegal cannabis products available, patients should know which are safe to vaporize. Some recreational cannabis concentrates, like vape cartridges, cannabis shatter, and cannabis wax, are designed for, and safe to use in, vaporizers, but these products are not currently legally available in Canada as either recreational or medical products. Though recreational legalization may spur change, the future availability of these products is still under some debate. Regardless, since most are high-THC products, they are not particularly useful for medical patients. In contrast to these cannabis concentrates designed for inhalational devices, the food-grade, ingestible oils offered by LPs are *never* safe to use in a vaporizer. These cannabinoid-infused oils are made with food-grade oils, like coconut or olive oils, and are intended for oral ingestion only. Vaporizing or smoking these ingestible oils is extremely dangerous. Inhaling their vapour or smoke can cause patients to develop lung disease, such as exogenous lipoid pneumonia, a serious illness that can even be fatal. Inhaling lipids and edible food oil into your lungs is toxic, dangerous, and damaging and should not be attempted.

Many vaporizer designs and models are available for patients to choose from. While this array of choices can seem confusing, broadly speaking there are only three main types: larger tabletop models, smaller portable models, and very small pen-sized varieties. However, most pen-style vaporizers, and some small portable models, are specifically designed for vaporizing the recreational cannabis concentrates discussed above. The only vaporizers a medical cannabis patient could currently use for dried medical cannabis are either tabletop or select portable varieties.

Tabletop Vaporizers

Tabletop vaporizers have the most advanced technology among vaporizers, with higher-end models offering significant precision and control over vaporizing temperatures and dose delivery. An example is the Volcano vaporizer, which can fill large medical-grade storage balloons, allowing delivery of multiple doses of medicine. Tabletop vaporizers are more suited to patients who primarily consume their cannabis at home and who are looking to get the most from their dried flower medicine. By controlling the exact temperature setting of the vaporizer, patients may help determine the cannabinoid profile they obtain, since each cannabinoid boils and vaporizes at a different temperature, allowing them to target individual cannabinoids and terpenes that they are receiving. Most high-end devices come with detailed instructions on how to target different cannabinoid profiles with different temperature settings. Unfortunately, the boiling points of the primary cannabinoids CBD and THC are similar, so separating these components by vaporizer adjustment is difficult.

Top-of-the-line advanced tabletop vaporizers tend to be quite expensive, and some research is likely warranted before purchase. These large vaporizers also need to be plugged into wall power and are not very portable. Therefore, they may not be the most economic or practical consumption method for most consumers.

Portable Vaporizers

For new medical cannabis patients who wish to find a practical, effective, and affordable option for their inhalational dosing regimen, the portable vaporizer is a good place to start. Once again, it's important to distinguish between vaporizers designed for concentrates and vaporizers designed for dried cannabis flower. As vaporizable concentrates are not legally available in Canada at the time of this writing, the latter type of vaporizer is the only option for medical cannabis patients in Canada. Also, remember that the cannabinoid oils that LPs sell are ingestible food oils, which are dangerous to vaporize and inhale, and so should never be used in a vaporizer.

As the market for cannabis continues to expand, so does the number and style of vaporizers. This wide variety can create some initial confusion for patients trying to decide which one of dozens of options is right for them. Portable vaporizers designed for dried flower are more complex than those designed for concentrates as they require a specific heating mechanism. This feature often makes them more expensive. Battery life is a major consideration for most patients, as are the vaporizer's overall efficiency, the ease of cleaning, and the presence of temperature controls. This information is complex enough that if a new patient is shopping for a vaporizer for medical cannabis purposes, it's helpful to go to a medical cannabis clinic with knowledgeable staff who can help to make that decision. Quality dried flower vaporizers are also likely going to be available at recreational outlets or online now that the Cannabis Act has passed.

Safety Concerns

Each available delivery mechanism has risks and benefits. Though I've already discussed some of the drawbacks of inhalation delivery methods, a brief but dedicated section is warranted to ensure prospective users are aware of risks. Smoking, of course, is not recommended. While direct links between cannabis smoking and lung cancer have never been proven, this risk is still theoretically present. Additionally, cannabis smokers frequently report respiratory symptoms, including coughing, wheezing, and airway irritation, and there appears to be increased risk of bronchitis and chronic pulmonary disease.

Existing data suggest that vaporizing cannabis is significantly less harmful than smoking cannabis. However, vaporizing is a relatively new delivery method, and no major randomized clinical trials have investigated long-term effects. Therefore, patients who choose to vaporize cannabis are accepting some unknown risk of this inhalational route of delivery, albeit much less than smoking as far as we know. Other risks of vaporizing include possible injuries from malfunction or overheating of the vaporizing device itself. In the recreational and nicotine vaporizing community, some awful burns and injuries have been reported. Most of these have come from malfunction of cheaply made recreational e-cigarette type devices. With quality controls in place for medical grade devices, risks of technical malfunction should be greatly reduced.

Other risks of inhalational use of cannabis are associated with the fact that it delivers the medical effect so quickly. The rapid and potentially intense onset of both therapeutic effects and side effects could cause impairment that might produce safety concerns, such as for patients who are driving vehicles, operating machinery, or risk falling. This danger is more common with inhalation of high-THC products. A final specific risk of inhalational delivery is accidental use of ingestible oils in a vaporizer. As discussed, the medical grade cannabis oils produced by LPs have an edible food-oil base and are dangerous and toxic to inhale. Vaporizing food oils produces lipid droplets that can be harmful to a patient's lungs.

ORAL DELIVERY METHODS

Oral delivery methods include any technique that administers cannabis through the mouth, such as tablets, gelcaps, tinctures, drops, and sprays for use under the tongue, and infused edible foods and drinks. Only one LP currently offers a sublingual spray formulation of its edible oil product, but under the Cannabis Act new oral formulations should be available soon. Edibles won't be available legally in Canada until at least October 2019, and then possibly only as recreational products. Because oils and gelcaps are currently the only oral medical products that LPs sell, much of our discussion will focus on them. Of course, some patients may choose to make their own edibles using available cannabis oils, so I'll also discuss those products as well.

Remember that ingested cannabis products typically have a slower onset and a longer-lasting effect than inhaled cannabis. This delayed onset can be a problem for new users who may keep taking more edible product thinking that it's not working, only to find they've taken too much medicine and then potentially experience effects, and possibly side effects, for hours. Therefore, patients who are cannabis naive and decide to use ingestible oils must follow health care provider recommendations carefully, start with the minimum amount, and titrate the dose incrementally and slowly. This caution is especially important for patients using high-THC oil as THC is the source of almost all cannabis-related side effects.

Ingestible Oils

Ingestible oils are typically sold in two primary forms, a liquid formulation designed to be delivered precisely with a dropper, and gelcaps containing precise quantities of the cannabis oil medicine. Both of these formulations look like conventional legitimate medicine to patients and providers, and consequently their popularity in Canada is growing compared with products for inhalation.

Besides allowing significant control over cannabinoid content and dosing, benefits of ingested oils are that they are discreet, easy to use, and versatile. The effects of a single dose can last up to eight hours, allowing a patient to medicate once in the morning and once in the evening in order to relieve symptoms throughout the day. And as already mentioned, the appearance and formulation of oils are consistent with conventional medicine, making these products more desirable for the medical consumer.

Since many traditional cannabis users think of cannabis based on weight as measured in grams, some patients would like to know exactly how much cannabis flower is in their medical oil. This idea is reinforced since the current medical document authorization is written in grams per day. Knowing exactly how much cannabis went into making a given volume of oil can be difficult as the conversion between dried flower and extract is complex and depends on many variables, and it's ultimately not as relevant as how much cannabinoid is present per millilitre of oil. Most simply, the conversion comes down to how many grams of dried plant product are required to produce a set amount of oil, and that will vary depending on manufacturing process and moisture content of the original plant material, among other factors. Most Canadian LPs have a conversion chart available. For example, one particular LP's oils all have an equivalency factor of 1 g dried cannabis to 5 mL cannabis oil. In that case, for ordering purposes, each 50 mL bottle of LP oil is equivalent to 10 grams of dried cannabis flower.

Unfortunately, the conversion factor often varies from one producer to another, so patients will need to check information provided by each LP on their website and on their product bottles.

Edibles

Edibles are any food or drink product containing cannabis. Another definition is food or beverage items that are infused with cannabis compounds. Up to this point, edibles have been illegal in Canada, but under the Cannabis Act they should be available after October 2019. In British Columbia, they have been widely available for years from unregulated dispensaries. They are a somewhat controversial topic when discussing medical cannabis since their use is often assumed to be recreational. However, they can provide an alternative to more conventional medical formulations. Typically, they provide effects similar to ingestible oils or gelcaps since they are also taken by mouth.

If patients are interested in edibles as a cannabis delivery method, they currently have to make them at home as medical cannabis edibles are not currently available from LPs. It's unclear if edible cannabis products will be integrated into the medical cannabis market. They will likely be available in recreational outlets in 2020, but these outlets are prohibited from selling medically specific phytocannabinoid products and are prohibited from providing specific medical advice. It's possible that cannabis edibles will never be formally introduced into the separate medical cannabis stream, although it's likely some medical patients will try them. Patients don't buy cookies infused with opiates or heart medicines from the pharmacy. A legitimate question is, should cannabis medicine be an exception?

Despite the debate about the legitimacy of edibles as a medical product, many Canadians have been self-medicating with homemade variants for years, often in the form of baked goods. Because plant cannabinoids dissolve in fats, they require a fat or oil base before being easily incorporated into foods. This fat solubility is why patients who make their own cannabis edibles from dried flower product often make cannabis butter first. LP-available oils can be used to make edibles directly since their bases are already food oils. Mixing known quantities of LP oil with other baking ingredients is likely the simplest way to make edibles at home. As mentioned, however, traditional homemade cannabis edibles are created by infusing a high-fat cooking ingredient, such as butter or olive oil, with cannabis. Some patients may also try to cook with whole dried cannabis flower without dissolving in an oil or fat base. Although this method is partially effective, it will usually make inefficient use of the medicine. Cannabinoids will activate unpredictably if cooked into edibles as raw plant material, and patients may find themselves using up a lot of expensive medicine for very little benefit. Patients who are particularly interested in cannabis edibles can find lots of recipes and information online. Generally speaking, becoming good at cooking with dried whole plant cannabis means perfecting the art of infusing cannabis into butter or oil.

Cooking with raw cannabis also requires a basic understanding of decarboxylation. Though I discussed the technical aspects of this process in Chapter 4, I'll mention a couple key points for those planning to make their own infused cannabis products. To decarboxylate at home, all you need is dried cannabis flower, an oven set to around 110°C (230°F), parchment paper, and a baking tray. Breaking the dried cannabis into small pieces, or using an official cannabis grinder, is important so it can be spread evenly and thinly over the baking sheet. Heat the cannabis in the oven for 45 minutes and the cannabinoids should be activated and ready for baking. Incorporation into butter usually involves pouring ground decarboxylated cannabis into butter, simmering for two to three hours, and then straining out plant fragments. Multiple recipes for this process are available online. An important caution: when baking in the oven, keep heat below 175°C (350°F) to avoid vaporizing off the cannabinoids. Most experienced patients who bake their own cannabis edibles keep the oven at 160°C (325°F). Since making cannabis edibles from scratch involves a fair amount of work, using edible oils from LPs can definitely speed up the process.

Safety Concerns

Oral ingestion of medicine also has its risks. Though unlikely, choking is a risk factor, particularly for patients who are weak or very ill and have trouble with airway protection. Another risk of oral cannabinoid ingestion is accidental ingestion, typically due to misinterpreting edibles as actual food. Edibles represent a particular risk of accidental consumption by children, particularly if they look like regular candies or treats. Therefore, cannabis edibles must be stored and labelled appropriately so that children, friends, or family don't accidentally consume them. They are also potentially dangerous to pets, who may be more sensitive to cannabis effects than their human counterparts.

Overconsumption of edibles is likely the biggest risk factor for ingestible cannabis medicine, usually due to taking more doses when effects are slow to initiate. Overconsumption is particularly problematic since the products may taste delicious, may look like standard food items, and have delayed effects. Since cannabis edibles have not yet been available within the legal Canadian medical cannabis market, these consumption concerns have not been major problems for medical cannabis patients. However, with rapid proliferation of recreational cannabis outlets and the new Cannabis Act's planned introduction of cannabis edibles in 2019, they may become more of an issue in the future.

If patients choose to consume cannabis edibles, or any oral cannabis product, they should be careful not to consume too much by adhering to the start-low, go-slow mantra discussed in Chapter 9. The advice to start with a very low dose of cannabis edibles is especially important if a patient is cannabis naive or is known to be sensitive to the psychoactive components of THC. Eating too many cannabis edibles can create an intense, and potentially very negative, experience. It may take two or three hours for ingested cannabinoids to fully absorb and activate in the body—a delayed onset that may prompt inexperienced or impatient consumers to eat more treats (like cookies, brownies, or gummy bears) in the interim. While overconsumption of cannabis edibles is not overtly dangerous and won't be permanently harmful or fatal, it can be so unpleasant that patients may believe they are going to die. It may temporarily incapacitate them, disrupting life activities and plans, and is generally a state worth avoiding. The best way to avoid excess cannabis edible ingestion is to ingest only regulated, licensed product of known composition and strength and carefully follow dosing recommendations (I provide guidelines in Chapter 9, though patients should adhere to their providers' advice).

If patients discover they have ingested too much THC, assuming that they have access and sufficient mental clarity, they should try ingesting a balanced dose of CBD. While this suggestion may sound like fighting fire with fire, as already mentioned, CBD counteracts the psychotropic effects of THC and has no impairing properties itself. If patients do not have access to CBD, they should try eating citrus fruits, pine nuts, or peppercorns. These foods contain terpenes known for increasing mental clarity and counteracting THC, including limonene, pinene, and caryophyllene.

TOPICAL DELIVERY METHODS

Until recently, most patients had never heard of topical cannabis preparations or the idea that cannabis medicine can be absorbed through the skin. However, most patients have heard of arthritis medicine that can be rubbed over sore joints that is absorbed for medical effect. Topical cannabis preparations work the same way to relieve localized symptoms, such as joint pain and inflammation, muscle aches and pains, or diseases of the skin. Topical application currently isn't a very popular way to use medical cannabis, and products haven't been widely available until recently. Currently, only one LP offers a kit for making a topical preparation from available oils, although introduction of pre-made topical preparations is pending under the Cannabis Act. These topical preparations are now gaining a lot of attention, particularly since new research is showing potential benefit for a number of conditions. Research is actively underway to determine the most absorbable and most effective topical cannabinoid preparations. These products currently include creams, oils, balms, and patches. Look for more information from LPs and cannabis clinics as new products are introduced.

While not widely studied, researchers have found that the topical application of cannabinoids usually has an onset of local action within minutes, with effects lasting approximately one to three hours. When used as directed to relieve localized symptoms, most topical cannabis users report an absence of psychoactive side effects and cite this as a major benefit of topicals. In fact, most topical cannabinoid medicine is absorbed into superficial tissues and does not significantly enter the bloodstream. Therefore, it's highly unlikely for the psychoactive compounds in cannabis to intoxicate users when applied topically, even for preparations containing THC. However, patients with topically treatable conditions, like skin disease or localized joint pain, who wish to avoid any risk of impairment may choose to use topical CBD-predominant cannabis. A possible exception to the non-intoxication of topically applied cannabinoids is a concentrated high-THC transdermal patch, which is an adhesive patch containing concentrated levels of medicine designed to be slowly absorbed through the skin and into the bloodstream. Although currently not legally available in Canada, the Cannabis Act will likely soon allow transdermal patch delivery of medical cannabis.

Safety Concerns

There aren't a lot of specific safety concerns when it comes to the topical application of cannabis medication, but a few potential issues are worth mentioning. The development of either a localized or more diffuse allergic reaction could occur with any topically applied medicine, in which case the medication should be washed off and discontinued. Localized skin irritation or worsening of an underlying skin condition could also occur. Patients should be careful not to touch their eyes after applying topical medication until they have washed their hands, as serious eye irritation could occur. Topical medication is meant to be applied in a small local area of the body. Rubbing the medicine diffusely all over the body increases risks of too much medication absorption and possible side effects.

SUPPOSITORIES

A suppository is a small, soft, rocket-shaped capsule that's designed to be inserted by the patient or caregiver through the anus. Suppositories are typically about an inch long and are made from a mixture of coconut oil, cocoa butter, or glycerin that is infused with cannabis or cannabis oil. Once inserted, the suppository dissolves and is absorbed into the bloodstream through the mucosal lining of the rectum. While some patients may be uncomfortable with the idea of inserting medicine into their anus, the lining of the rectum absorbs many medicines well, and rectal cannabis administration has potential benefits.

The primary indications for using suppositories are in patients who can't take medications by mouth. These cases include patients with severe nausea and vomiting, patients with active convulsions, patients who are confused or agitated, and patients who are not allowed to eat and drink for various reasons (like surgery or trauma). For patients with chemotherapy-induced nausea and vomiting who are too sick to ingest or inhale anything by mouth, suppositories can be the only available way to take cannabis. They are also helpful in patients with facial injuries, oral ulcerations, or any other condition limiting ability to take medications orally or by inhalation. Because the onset and duration of rectal cannabis suppositories is typically slow and prolonged, similar to the absorption and action of cannabis edibles, suppositories can also be an ideal treatment option for palliative patients who need long-lasting background symptom relief but are unable to take medicine orally due to weakness or choking risk.

One of the theoretical benefits of rectal cannabis delivery is that some of the rectally absorbed medicine goes to body tissues directly without metabolism by the liver. Medicine absorbed by the GI tract normally goes to the liver first, but some medicines absorbed through the rectum bypass the liver due to rectal venous anatomy. This pathway is known medically as *bypass of first-pass hepatic metabolism* and could, in theory, make rectally administered cannabis medicine more bioavailable than cannabis delivered by other means. In reality, suppositories enter through the anal canal but sit up in the rectum where middle and upper rectal veins drain. Therefore, much of the cannabis medicine absorption primarily goes through the portal venous system and does not bypass the liver. At least some medicine is likely quickly absorbed in the lower rectum and does bypass first-pass metabolism, but the clinical benefits are questionable. Although this type of absorption would theoretically allow for greater bioavailability, in general most rectal absorption is slow, and the total rate and extent of rectal absorption tends to actually be lower than that seen with oral delivery. In other words, the overall mechanism of drug absorption from the rectum is probably not substantially different from that in the upper part of the GI tract. Suppositories therefore offer no major clinical benefits other than administration in patients who can't use the oral route.

Rectal administration also has some disadvantages. First is the fact that it requires inserting something into the anus, which for some people is physically difficult, uncomfortable, and not an appealing idea. Second is the fact that the rectum is a storage organ for fecal material. Inserting a suppository into a rectum full of stool can trigger a bowel movement, which flushes out the suppository. Feces in the rectum can seriously interfere with medicine absorption as well. Overall, I suspect that rectal suppository administration has enough downsides that its potential benefits are not worthwhile for most medical cannabis patients. For the same reasons, rectal administration of conventional pharmaceuticals is not very common or popular.

A final point to keep in mind is that, in general, putting a medicine close to an area of pain isn't as successful as good systemic absorption. That is why, for example, most menstrual cramp and prostate medicines are taken by mouth rather than inserted in the vagina or put up the penis. Similarly, there is no evidence that cannabis suppositories are any better for low back pain, menstrual cramps, or other local pain than oral or inhaled cannabis. There is also currently no evidence that cannabis suppositories combat rectal or prostate cancers. These diseases are treated with systemic chemotherapy and local radiation.

Safety Concerns

The primary risk of rectal administration is inadvertent injury to the anorectal area during insertion of a suppository. This area of the body is extremely vascular, and a common manifestation of injury might be exacerbation of hemorrhoidal type bleeding. While the suppository itself is soft and unlikely to cause harm, a fingernail or foreign body could cause injury. The second primary risk of rectal administration is the triggering of a bowel movement, which could cause discomfort or social embarrassment. Finally, like oral administration, rectal administration has slow onset and prolonged effects so the results of using too much medication could be unpleasant and last many hours.

CHAPTER 12
REGULATIONS AND SAFETY

It has been a slow process coming to where we are in Canada today with regard to cannabis regulations. Even now, seventeen years since Canadians were granted access to legal medical cannabis, the regulations are still evolving. Underlying this slow process is the goal of respecting the rights of Canadians to access clean, safe, regulated medical cannabis while maintaining an emphasis on community well-being and public safety.

PURCHASE, POSSESSION, AND STORAGE OF CANNABIS

Under the Cannabis Act, any Canadian eighteen years or older (as defined by rules in each province) has the legal right to purchase up to 30 g of cannabis at a time from a provincially regulated cannabis outlet, whether it be online or storefront. They are also able to possess or share up to 30 g of cannabis in public. Personal storage limits for cannabis have been removed, and Canadians may now store an unlimited amount of personal-use cannabis at home.

In addition to their rights under the Cannabis Act, medical patients under the revised ACMPR rules are still allowed to purchase medical cannabis from LPs using a signed medical document from a health care provider. With proof of status as a medical patient, the maximum amount of cannabis a medical patient is allowed to possess publicly is 150 g in addition to the 30 g recreational limit. Patients in public possession of more than the 30 g recreational limit of cannabis product will be expected to prove their status as a legitimate medical patient to law enforcement if requested. Proof may be demonstrated by providing a registration document issued by a federally licensed seller, a registration certificate issued by Health Canada for personal or designated production, or a new registration certificate issued by Health Canada for medical possession only. The new Cannabis Act eliminates private possession and storage limits at home for medical patients as well. Storage requirements for medical cannabis are similar to those for other prescription medications. Storage is recommended to be in areas not easily accessible by children and ideally in childproof medication containers.

TRAVELLING WITH CANNABIS

Since there has been such a rapid and radical shift in attitudes toward cannabis, many patients have understandable concerns about the legalities of travelling with their medicine. Both the ACMPR and the Cannabis Act are federal laws, which apply anywhere within Canada. Patients have had the legal right to travel with authorized medical cannabis anywhere in the country since 2013. Now, all adult Canadians have the same legal rights with regard to transporting recreational cannabis within the public possession limits. It's legal to transport cannabis on airplanes, buses, trains, and rapid transit. Local authorities and transport security are legally bound to accept and support a Canadian's right to do so, as long as the travel is within this country. When travelling by plane, it's recommended to keep medical cannabis in carry-on luggage since checked luggage can go missing and theft of medication from luggage does occur. For patients travelling with liquid cannabis preparations, the 100 mL maximum liquid allowance will still apply. If travelling with more than the 30 g recreational allotment, patients must be prepared to prove that that they are legal medical cannabis patients.

To prove status as a medical patient, I advise that medical cannabis is kept in the original container it arrived in from the LP. All of the relevant prescription details (including prescribing health care provider, prescribed period of use, and patient name, among others), will be printed on the container. Until recently, this packaging was the only way of legitimizing possession of any cannabis in Canada. With the new Cannabis Act in force, I recommend that medical patients carrying more than the 30 g recreational limit also travel with proof of being a medical cannabis patient, as detailed in the previous section.

Remember that although both patients and recreational users may travel with ease in Canada while possessing cannabis, this allowance does not apply beyond our borders. The laws in Canada are in direct contrast with the laws in the United States, presenting potential risk to Canadians who are travelling south of the border. Currently, every US state has a different set of laws regarding cannabis. Despite legal status in some states, the US federal government continues to classify cannabis as an illegal Schedule I drug. At a federal level, there is still rigid enforcement of cannabis possession laws, and the border is under federal jurisdiction. Canadians travelling to Washington State, or other states where cannabis is also legal, often assume that keeping cannabis in their possession is okay. This is absolutely not true. Officers at US entries along the Canadian border enforce all federal laws, and cannabis possession is strictly prohibited. Recently, a number of unwitting Canadian business travellers have received lifetime bans from the United States simply for admitting to working full time in the cannabis industry. While those decisions may ultimately be reversed, violating US drug policy at the border can have serious and long-lasting consequences. Possessing cannabis, using cannabis, or making a living from the sale of cannabis is a federal crime in the US. As long as cannabis remains a Schedule I drug in the US, great care must be taken not to inadvertently violate these laws. Do not attempt to cross any US border while in possession of cannabis, whether it's medical or not.

Few international nations agree on how to deal with the issue of medical cannabis during travel, and the laws that constitutionally support access to cannabis in Canada are not recognized in other countries. While agreements between countries allowing travel with medical cannabis are likely to develop in the future, crossing any international border with cannabis is strongly discouraged. It's also important to remember that, just like any regular medical prescription, your medical cannabis document is specific to Canada and can't be used internationally. Therefore, patients can't use their Canadian document to buy medical cannabis in countries that have a legal system for authorized medical cannabis of their own.

DRIVING SAFETY

The primary factor when considering driving safety is whether medical cannabis use causes dangerous driving. Impaired driving is unacceptable, dangerous, and illegal. Substance-related impaired driving is a major cause of injury and death in North America, and studies repeatedly show that alcohol and drugs are major contributing factors to a large number of fatal motor vehicle accidents.[262] Motor vehicle accidents remain a leading cause of accidental death and disability worldwide. In Canada, the percentage of drivers killed in vehicle crashes who test positive for drugs (40 percent) now exceeds the percentage who test positive for alcohol (33 percent).[263]

Statistics

In both 2017 and 2018, Health Canada conducted a survey of self-reported cannabis-use patterns in Canada, which included an assessment of cannabis use in relation to driving.[264,265] Driving after using cannabis specifically for medical purposes was studied among respondents. Of respondents, 37 percent in 2017 and 40 percent in 2018 reported that they had driven within two hours of using cannabis for medical purposes. In both years, male patients (46 percent) were more likely to report driving within two hours of using cannabis for medical purposes than female patients (28 percent). Therefore, it appears that a significant number of patients are driving after taking medical cannabis. Since the survey didn't identify the type of medical products taken by patients, it's difficult to estimate risk of impairment. Of more potential concern was that 10 percent of respondents indicated that they had driven a vehicle within two hours of using cannabis for medical purposes in combination with alcohol.

Research and Regulations

The data and statistics for cannabis-specific related motor vehicle accidents are mixed, at best. Unfortunately, despite the blood levels stated below, there is no agreed upon blood level of cannabis that separates impaired from non-impaired drivers. However, due to known effects of THC on concentration and motor function, legislators have identified the need for defining legal THC limits. Currently, in most North American jurisdictions, the accepted standard for safe driving is a blood THC level of less than 5 ng/mL, and this concentration level was originally proposed as the legal limit in Canada.

In the end, new drug-impaired driving legislation came into force in Canada June 21, 2018, and the legislation created three new offences for having a prohibited concentration of THC in the blood within two hours of driving. The blood THC levels were set at 2 to 5 ng/mL for a summary conviction of up to a $1,000 fine, 5 ng/mL or greater for a mandatory minimum $1,000 fine, and a hybrid offense for drivers who consumed both cannabis and alcohol presenting with a blood alcohol concentration of 50 mg alcohol per 100 mL blood and a blood THC concentration of at least 2.5 ng/mL for a mandatory minimum $1,000 fine. All offenses other than a summary conviction carry minimum mandatory imprisonment of at least thirty days after the first offense.

While these limits may be the new law, the difficulty is that multiple studies have questioned the validity of the 5 ng/mL measure. An as-yet-unpublished trial from the University of British Columbia showed no statistical association with impairment at a blood level of 5 ng/mL and only mild association at higher blood levels. Unfortunately, some cannabis users are impaired with less than 5 ng/mL blood level while others show no impairment at a much higher level. Additionally, regular users will often test positive days after any possible impairing effects of the drug have worn off. However, the new laws are in place and users of THC need to realize that punishments are severe, particularly for repeat offenders.

Some of the new blood THC concentration limits will likely be tested in court, particularly since they don't correlate with impairment. The Canadian government has admitted this and stated that the established levels were based on a precautionary approach. Ideally, rather than an arbitrary blood level, which is not based on scientific studies, we should really be concerned with keeping impaired drivers off the road. How to do this fairly and accurately is the big question. Any amount of any substance that causes impairment of concentration or reduced motor coordination and reaction time is unacceptable from a public safety standpoint.

The reality, however, is that we all accept the risks inherent in driving on common over-the-counter cold or anti-nausea medications that produce sedation and delayed reaction. We also accept the risks of people driving home tired after long, exhausting days or nights at work. Neither of these examples have validated roadside impairment or blood tests available. What cannabis driving enforcement will likely come down to are enhanced field sobriety and impairment testing performed by police officers who observe impaired driving behaviour. The blood testing would then be a back-up for observed impaired driving behaviour. Police groups are currently studying modifications to field sobriety tests that might be more sensitive to cannabis impairment.[266]

Cannabis and Other Inebriants

In determining the degree to which cannabis use contributes to motor vehicle collisions, another factor is the presence of additional or confounding inebriants. The majority of drivers involved in fatal accidents who test positive for cannabis also test positive for alcohol or other recreational drugs. While studies confirm that alcohol impairment is much more dangerous than cannabis impairment, the combination of the two has been shown to be more dangerous than either drug separately.[267] An additional study of motor vehicle crash risk initially found a statistically significant increase in crash risk for drivers who tested positive for THC specifically. However, after adjusting for age and alcohol concentration, they did not find a significant increase in crash risk associated with cannabis use alone.[268] Therefore, the confounding effects of alcohol and cannabis together must be considered, and the associated risk is one reason that Canadian law prohibits alcohol and cannabis sales occurring at the same business or in close proximity. It's also the reason that new impaired driving laws in Canada give harsh penalties for the combination of alcohol and THC.

The *Canadian Cannabis Survey* asked respondents who indicated they had driven within two hours of using cannabis if they drove a vehicle within two hours of using cannabis in combination with alcohol.[264] Fifteen percent of the recreational respondents and 10 percent of the medical respondents reported that they had. The same respondents were also asked if they drove a vehicle within two hours of using cannabis in combination with other drugs. Eight percent of these respondents reported that they had. A firm message has to be communicated that cannabis use in combination with other drugs or alcohol may produce a dangerous and illegal impairment of driving ability. Such use is both morally and legally unacceptable for anyone who chooses to get behind the wheel of a motor vehicle while so impaired.

Duration of Impairment

Patients often ask how long after they use cannabis medicine are they safe to drive. As both recreational and medical cannabis become increasingly available, it will be extremely important to know the answer to this question. Deciding when and if a driver is legally impaired can have immense ramifications in the event of an accident. While law enforcement and the courts have been able to establish a stable system for determining intoxication in cases of alcohol intake, the same is not necessarily true for cannabis and particularly not for cannabis medicine. The THC in cannabis is what produces impairment, but THC content varies immensely depending on the type of cannabis a person is using. THC is also known to affect people dramatically differently depending on their tolerance levels and many other variables. While we continue to develop sensible cannabis policy as it relates to driving, the take-home message is that no impairment is acceptable when operating a motor vehicle. This hard rule is obviously difficult to follow since our current reality already includes non-cannabis–related variables, such as fatigue, medical conditions, visual acuity, cell phones, and other driver distractions.

Currently, the generic recommendation from Health Canada states that no one should drive or operate machinery for three to four hours after inhaling cannabis or for six to eight hours after ingesting cannabis. The Canadian Armed Forces have set twenty-four hours as the time a service member can operate a vehicle after using any form of cannabis, while some provincial law enforcement groups have set the time as twenty-eight days. Until we get better science and studies of actual impairment with specific medical cannabis products, we are likely to see this sort of wide variation in rules and recommendations. Remember that while using cannabis medicine is legal, impaired driving is not.

CANNABIS AT WORK

Almost all employers have established workplace safety protocols and guidelines in place. Large corporations specializing in areas with significant public safety concerns, such as petroleum, mining, construction, and airline industries, have particularly detailed policies. Ultimately, however, all medicines, including over-the-counter medicines, have potential side effects, and it's the employee who is obligated not to work while impaired. Due to safety concerns, some employers have zero-tolerance policies for certain medications. When starting any new medication, it's always wise for employees to err on the side of caution. This warning is particularly true for cannabis medicine since employee guidelines are still evolving. An example of a current grey area is CBD-based medication. Evidence suggests that pure CBD oil is not functionally impairing and theoretically would not interfere with ability to work or drive. However, even "pure" CBD preparations often have trace amounts of THC, which could show up on roadside testing or workplace drug monitoring programs. Ultimately, it's up to patients to follow their employers' policies with regard to the use of cannabis medicine.

Worker Rights and Responsibilities

Since 2001, Canadians have had the legal right to use medical cannabis as they would use any other medication. Under current regulations, patients must obtain specific medical cannabis products only from a government-regulated LP or distributor and only after they have obtained a recommendation and signed medical document from a licensed health care provider. In this way, authorization for use comes directly from the patients' health care provider. Therefore, workplace standards and guidelines should ultimately address the use of medical cannabis in the same way that internal policies deal with other prescribed pharmaceuticals. Workplace standards with regard to recreational cannabis will likely follow the same internal policies as those addressing alcohol.

Often, standard medication policies require the patient to follow a health care provider's strict instructions with regard to dosing and frequency of use. Unfortunately, cannabis science does not currently provide enough evidence to dictate a strict regimen for frequency and dosage of medical use, and the current ACMPR law does not allow providers to stipulate these parameters on the medical document. Additionally, multiple formulations and varieties of medical cannabis products are available, some of which could cause impairment and others not. Medical providers currently have no legal control over which products patients purchase or use once medical authorization for cannabis is given. Therefore, individual medical cannabis use, and side effects of such use, vary tremendously from one patient to another. This variability makes development of standardized workplace compliance rules regarding cannabis more difficult than for most other pharmaceuticals. For this reason, workplace policies may vary quite markedly from one employer to another.

While patients have the constitutional legal right to use medical cannabis in Canada, they do not have the right to be impaired at work. While the employer is obligated to make allowances for patients to use legal, non-impairing medicines at work, the employee is obligated to follow specific workplace guidelines regarding safety and impairment. The difficulty arises when an employer's zero-tolerance cannabis policy clashes with a worker's right to use non-impairing medicine. Ultimately, validated studies looking at the effects of various medical cannabis products on work performance, motor coordination, and cognitive ability will be needed to resolve these is-sues. Many of these questions may also be answered in the Canadian courts after inevitable legal challenges arise.

In fact, some legal precedents and protections for patients have already developed from legal proceedings. In 2015, an Alberta arbitra-tion board ruled in favour of an employee when his company relieved him of a safety-sensitive position (operating a grader on city streets) after admitting to cannabis use. The grader operator confessed to tak-ing small amounts of cannabis at night before bed, to address his back pain, and the City of Calgary (his employer) elected to remove him from his position. The board of arbitration ordered an indepen-dent medical investigation, and, based on the evidence (notably, zero evidence of substance abuse or impairment at work), ordered the man be reinstated to his former position.

As cannabis legislation evolves and matures across Canada, at-titudes toward cannabis will change, and research on the effects of cannabis in a variety of work-related scenarios will be conducted. Because medical cannabis use is still considered controversial by some, I recommend that patients discuss legitimate medical use with their employers. Under the Canadian Human Rights Act, employers are obligated to eliminate negative treatment of individuals based on prohibited grounds of discrimination, including medical disability. Therefore, employers are legally required to meet these human rights obligations toward employees with medical conditions who need to take health care provider–authorized cannabis medication. This ob-ligation does not override workplace policy on impairment-related safety issues, however. Although medical cannabis authorization doesn't allow a patient to smoke in a non-smoking area, employers must accommodate users of any prescribed inhaled or injectable med-icines to take breaks to administer medicines in suitable areas. For workers in safety-sensitive positions, temporary reassignment may be needed until they are deemed fully fit to return to duty. Incidents like the unwarranted termination of the employee in Calgary are be-coming rare, and companies are increasingly becoming proactive in developing accommodating medical cannabis policies that don't com-promise their safety standards.

Safety Concerns and Regulations

The NAS review on the health effects of cannabis reviewed six studies published since 1999 on cannabis use and workplace injury.[72] These studies assessed only recreational cannabis use as widespread use of medical cannabis products in the workplace has become common only recently. The NAS reviewers concluded that there is currently "insufficient evidence to support or refute a statistical association between general, non-medical cannabis use and occupational accidents or injuries." In other words, at this time we do not have enough data to assess the workplace effects of cannabis in general and specifically the effects of medical cannabis products. Despite lack of scientific evidence, widespread use of cannabis products in the workplace does raise a number of potentially legitimate safety concerns for employers. In safety-sensitive work positions, impairment could lead to significant disability or loss of life, not only to the employee but to others. Safety-sensitive work positions are defined as those that, if not performed in a safe manner, can cause direct and significant damage to property, and/or injury to the employee, others around them, the public and/or the immediate environment.

Currently, there is an absence of consistent federal, provincial, and territorial legislation concerning cannabis consumption and workplace safety. Employers across Canada are struggling to balance the need to protect their employees' rights with the need to maintain a safe work environment. Employees are equally confused, wondering whether small doses of non-impairing CBD oil will cost them their jobs or when (if ever) to discuss their cannabis prescription with their employers. Because health care providers are not authorized by the ACMPR to dictate product types or dosing to patients via the medical document, it's not possible for a medical cannabis provider to make specific recommendations or assessments with regard to workplace safety. Each employer must follow their own policies and procedures when it comes to safety issues.

From a safety standpoint, employers will consider numerous factors, but the ultimate question is related to the presence or absence of impairment. As with any prescription medication, employees are usually deemed unfit for work if they are impaired by a medication.

Multiple existing prescription and non-prescription medicines are known to cause impairment, and current workplace safety guidelines are in place to address their use. In terms of risk assessment, each employer must address safety-sensitive work issues relating to a worker's use of any medication, including cannabis. Should a fitness-for-duty medical examination be required, it should be performed by a specialist in occupational safety and medicine.

From an alcohol- and drug-testing perspective, users of medical cannabis may or may not test positive for cannabis use due to the lack of available tests for some forms of cannabis medicine. Additionally, chronic users of medical cannabis may test positive on urine or blood tests days or weeks after last known use. These delayed positive tests can be explained by the slow breakdown and fat solubility of cannabis metabolites, and they remain an unresolved issue in the development of fair drug testing protocols for cannabis medicine. Unlike alcohol, no specific laboratory tests accurately predict impaired function with cannabis. There is no set blood level that has been proven to demonstrate whether a patient is fit or not for safe work. This uncertainty remains a significant challenge for cannabis medicine.

Ultimately, it's the responsibility of each employer to follow existing internal policy, and it's not within the purview or ability of health care providers to determine if an individual medical cannabis patient is fit for work. It is, however, reasonable for health care providers to inform patients who are receiving a new medical document authorizing cannabis that all medicines have the potential to cause impairment, that they are responsible for following their employers' workplace and safety rules, and that some employers have a zero-THC testing policy. Being an authorized user of legal medical cannabis does not give a patient the right to ignore workplace safety rules. On the other hand, authorized users of medical cannabis have all the rights and protections afforded to users of other prescription medications.

Impairment Concerns and Job Performance

Although safety is the primary concern when it comes to cannabis use in the workplace, employers are also concerned about other impairment-related factors, including tardiness and absenteeism, decreased cognitive performance, and reduced efficiency. More than three hundred thousand Canadians are already active medical cannabis users, the majority of whom are work-age adults. Therefore, medical cannabis use at work is a real issue. Medical cannabis patients must understand both patient rights and responsibilities with regard to cannabis in the workplace. As mentioned above, policies regarding safety and compliance vary from one employer to another, with the basic understanding that impairment is not acceptable and that all workplace rules must be followed.

So how do we approach the question, will cannabis-based therapy affect job performance? The same question could be applied to cold medicines, antidepressants, or other commonly used medications. We usually accept the workplace effects of medication if the positive benefits outweigh any negative effects. The drowsiness of cold medicines is accepted if they allow you to feel better, get out of bed, and carry on with normal activities of daily living. However, the truth is that users of over-the-counter cold medicines are often drowsy at work, and that drowsiness may affect their work performance. It's hard to draw a clear line between impaired and unimpaired with regard to use of medications in the workplace as the interpretation is often subjective. In terms of cannabis medicine, a patient may find that far from being impaired, taking cannabis has enabled them to work pain-free with sharper focus, and their employer may agree. However, if that same employee were evaluated by an objective drug test analysis, the results might give a different definition of impairment.

As already mentioned, drug testing for cannabis is far from an exact science, and existing tests have many known problems. It's widely acknowledged that the margin for error on these tests is high, generating many false negatives and false positives due to the length of time cannabis may remain in the human body. Unfortunately, positive blood tests for cannabis do not correlate with actual impairment. Because cannabis metabolites are fat soluble and are stored in the body, they may be detectable in blood tests for days or weeks after last medical use. That delayed detection makes the use of cannabis medicine by patients in zero-tolerance positions very difficult or impossible. I expect that many of these work regulations will be challenged in court, which will likely spur us to develop more refined testing and policies that actually address impairment rather than arbitrary blood tests that may or may not indicate a true impairment issue.

Unfortunately, research is way behind on studying the effects of individual cannabinoids with respect to dosage and side effects. We know a lot about how many medicines work under a wide variety of circumstances, but the many variables of medical cannabis make our ability to predict the plant's effects on individual users quite challenging. While one person may be rendered impaired by a small dose of cannabis, another may not notice any effects from an even larger dose of medicine. We know from existing driving safety studies that some heavy chronic cannabis users do not show evidence of impairment despite high blood levels of THC.[269] These drivers did not demonstrate any objective driving impairment. Meanwhile, some novice cannabis users become impaired with very small doses of cannabis. Keep in mind that these data are from the use of recreational high-THC cannabis. We do not have significant data on whether medical cannabis products, like CBD-predominant preparations, cause functional impairment, although data we have suggests they do not. These realities make generation of sensible cannabis policy challenging.

While there are no easy answers, it should be possible to arrive at reasonable guidelines by continuing to explore and discuss the issue. Cannabis medicine is just medicine, and employers deal with their employees taking medicines every day. Each workplace is different, and each will likely have a different policy regarding the use of medicines, including cannabis. In safety-sensitive employment sectors, including oil, mining, construction, transportation, health care, and law enforcement, employers will be very cautious regarding medication use and will have testing protocols in place to ensure safety. Other work environments will likely be more permissive. Ultimately, however, employers understandably expect their employees to be able to successfully complete their work each day, unimpaired by the effects of their medicine. With that goal, employers' expectations are in line with the intent of health care providers, which is to relieve symptoms without interfering with normal function.

USING CANNABIS UNDER SPECIAL CIRCUMSTANCES

Since cannabis is now legal both medically and recreationally, its use will become common in everyday life in Canada. Medical cannabis patients will use cannabis within specific facilities, like nursing homes or hospitals, and under special circumstances, such as before and after surgery. I briefly discuss some of these particular situations below.

In a Hospital Setting

Hospitals across Canada are starting to develop specific cannabis-use policies to address the new status of cannabis as a legitimate legal medicine. This process is often made easier by taking existing alcohol and non-formulary medication policy and adapting it to apply to cannabis. Challenges remain, including integration of cannabis medicine into the electronic medical record and provider order-entry systems. Therefore, patients should expect that they may need to work collaboratively with their care teams to make continued use of their cannabis medicine possible within the hospital setting. When being admitted to hospital, patients should be open with health care workers regarding their status as medical cannabis patients and outline their anticipated needs for cannabis consumption during the hospital stay.

Currently, a number of potential barriers to consuming cannabis in a hospital setting persist. First, inhaling cannabis may violate existing no-smoking policies. There will be concerns about the possibility of second-hand smoke or vapour and the effects on other patients and staff. Most hospital campuses are now smoke free due to known health risks of cigarette smoking. Policies around vaporizing are usually in line with smoking policies, and using dried cannabis by inhalation is not currently allowed in most hospitals. With the expected development of cannabis nebulizers and asthma style inhalers, patients will likely be able to inhale cannabis medicine in hospitals with more ease soon.

Second, if a patient is too sick or incapacitated to administer cannabis on their own, there may still be some legal and procedural ambiguity regarding the health care team's ability to assist with medication delivery. Preparing the cannabis and arriving at a specific dose can be a time-consuming process, and the lack of defined dosing and frequency data for cannabis can clash with a regimented conventional hospital model where medications are usually delivered at strict intervals in secure packaging. Medical cannabis patients are often involved with every step of their medication delivery. When incapacitated in hospital, the needs of the medical cannabis patient may create added work and responsibilities for an already-busy health care team, and those needs may or may not be accommodated. Hospital pharmacies are typically not equipped with cannabis products or medical devices that administer cannabis, which means if a patient wishes to continue using cannabis during a hospital stay, and the hospital permits use, they may need to bring their own medical products and devices. Use of home medication and devices may or may not be possible depending on individual hospital policy.

If a patient expresses a desire to use cannabis during their hospital stay but policy doesn't allow use of home medications, health care providers may recommend a temporary switch to an approved pharmaceutical cannabinoid, such as a synthetic THC, like nabilone, or a balanced THC–CBD product, like nabiximols. In the near future, many hospital pharmacies may also start to carry Epidiolex, a pharmaceutical CBD preparation. These products are considered standard prescription medicines and are increasingly carried in hospital pharmacies. Using a standard pharmaceutical allows the hospital and its care team to dispense, administer, and regulate the medication based on conventional medication guidelines, and eliminates the barriers that would be involved if a patient continued to self-administer their own supply of cannabis medicine.

Due to the amazing variety of currently available recreational and medical cannabis products, it's not possible for hospitals to approve and dispense them all. Therefore, pharmaceutical cannabinoid medicines, like nabilone, nabiximols, and Epidiolex, may ultimately be the only available substitutes for herbal cannabis in the event of surgery or hospitalization. It's not common, but some patients who are regular cannabis users suffer from unpleasant symptoms if they suddenly stop using cannabis. This cannabis withdrawal syndrome is increasingly being recognized and often manifests as irritability, difficulty sleeping, and GI upset. While not overtly dangerous, like the withdrawal from opiates, benzodiazepines, or alcohol, these symptoms can make a hospital stay even more difficult. Therefore, if patients have previously experienced, or feel at risk of developing, cannabis withdrawal symptoms, they should notify their health care team. Studies have shown that nabiximols and other pharmaceutical cannabinoid preparations can help prevent and treat cannabis withdrawal.[270] Therefore, even if herbal cannabis is not approved in the hospital, usually some means of accommodating medical cannabis needs can be found.

Before or After Surgery
No major trials have evaluated the safety or efficacy of cannabis used before or shortly after surgery, so I therefore encourage caution. Generally speaking, the acute intoxicating effects of recreational cannabis use will wear off within a few hours, so regular pre-operative precautions, such as no smoking within three to four hours before surgery and nothing by mouth after midnight, will offer adequate protection against most risks. Smoking cannabis can increase coughing, sputum production, and respiratory secretions. These effects could interfere with airway protection and breathing during surgery and therefore should be avoided completely to maximize peri-operative safety. Acute cannabis intoxication can alter heart rate, increase or decrease blood pressure, or possibly exacerbate anaesthetic pharmaceutical effects. Additionally, cannabis intoxication can interfere with bispectral index monitoring, which is an indicator of depth of anaesthesia.[271] Therefore, patients needing urgent surgery who are intoxicated with cannabis must be honest with their surgeon and anaesthesiologist. In addition to potential interference with monitoring, regular heavy cannabis use may also affect how much anaesthesia medication is required, so being truthful about chronic use is also important.

Post-operatively, smoking any compound is discouraged, both to alleviate risks of second-hand smoke on other patients and to lessen post-operative respiratory risks. Cannabis smoking is also associated with fits of violent coughing in some patients, which could disrupt wounds or healing surgical sites. Therefore, I do not recommend post-operative cannabis smoking. Data on potential benefit of using post-operative oral or vaporized cannabis products are not currently available since the research hasn't been conducted. There is, however, some increasing evidence of opiate-sparing effects of cannabis in chronic pain, and some anecdotal reports of the same opiate-sparing potential in post-operative patients (refer to Chapter 8 for more information on these effects). Therefore, it's possible that cannabis medicines may eventually be incorporated into post-surgical care. Hopefully, research will validate these effects and allow development of therapeutic pathways that include safe cannabis delivery as part of the post-operative treatment plan.

In a Hospice or Assisted-Living Setting

For an in-patient at a hospice facility or one who resides at a long-term care home or an assisted-living community, accessing cannabis or having it administered may present challenges. To begin with, it may be difficult to arrange an initial assessment by a cannabis-educated health care provider in order to acquire a medical document and then register with an LP. If the patient experiences significant transfer and mobility issues, visiting a medical cannabis specialist may not be possible. In this case, it may be possible to send a legal proxy using personal health directive instructions. Caregivers signify their legal rights as patient representatives for medical issues by obtaining and providing a valid, signed personal directive document. For decision making over payment or financial matters related to the medical cannabis purchase, the caregiver would also need a signed power of attorney document. The medical clinic will likely need to examine the legal proxy documents prior to proceeding with an appointment.

Registering with an LP almost always requires using a computer, tablet, or phone with access to the internet, another complication for many older or institutionalized patients. Finally, once these patients have their cannabis medication, simply preparing and consuming the cannabis may be challenging—no matter what consumption method is chosen. These barriers often leave patients totally reliant on their health care teams, and the standards of practice governing nurses' and care professionals' ability to administer cannabis are still evolving. Standards and guidelines are often different from one province to another, and in many jurisdictions there remain many unanswered questions. Ultimately, it's up to each province, municipality, and institution to develop and implement a sensible medical cannabis policy. This will take time, but already guidelines and regulations are being developed and refined.

WHEN NOT TO USE CANNABIS

As stressed throughout this book, one of the most remarkable and best things about cannabis is its amazing safety profile. There are very few contraindications for any cannabis product, and despite being used by people with nearly every medical condition imaginable, there have been no documented medical cannabis–related deaths. Still, use of cannabis medicine is not suitable in a number of situations.

Prospective patients with one of the relative contraindications discussed in Chapter 5 should not receive authorized cannabis from a health care provider in Canada unless benefits of therapy clearly outweigh risks. Patients working in jobs with zero-THC policies may choose to use another form of medication until newer cannabis-use policy is developed. Most importantly, patients should not take any cannabis medicine that might cause impairment if they are driving or working in safety-sensitive positions.

While we know from experience and preliminary data that CBD is non-impairing, currently available cannabis use recommendations are all grouped together. Therefore, formal recommendations that apply to cannabis should be generally applied to all forms of cannabis medicine since there are currently no separate contraindications, guidelines, or recommendations for CBD or other specific medicinal cannabis products. With research and time, we'll be in a position to make more specific and refined recommendations regarding the use of a variety of cannabis medicine products in a range of life and work circumstances.

PART V
THE FUTURE OF MEDICAL CANNABIS

In Canada, after a century of prohibition and stigmatization, we have finally arrived at a place of common sense, where cannabis may be used legally both as a medicine and as a recreational euphoriant and relaxant. We have passed the point where use of a legitimate pharmacological medicine is discouraged or prohibited, and hopefully no one else will lose a life or livelihood due to possession or use of a natural compound that is certainly safer than alcohol. For the author of this book, someone who wrote their high school paper on why cannabis should be legalized almost forty years ago, this change is a long time coming and significant vindication.

The fact that cannabis can be used safely and effectively both recreationally and medicinally is a unique situation, which does create some challenges. Is a dried cannabis flower medicine, a recreational product, or both? Where is the line between recreational and medical use? I would argue that due to the incredible safety profile of cannabis, at some level it doesn't matter. I would also argue that the intention of the user helps to answer the question. And finally, I would argue that we are heading toward a situation where recreational and medicinal cannabis products are, for the most part, completely different. Not only will the branding and packaging look different, but the products themselves will also have completely different chemical profiles and intended effects. The goal of medical therapy is relief of symptoms without impairment. The goal of recreational use is relaxation, euphoria, and enhancement of reality without personal or community harm. In either situation, when used appropriately cannabis can be a significant positive, resulting in increased enjoyment, enhanced well-being, and improved quality of life.

Whole plant cannabis is a marvellously complex natural product. Hundreds of chemical compounds exist within one plant, and the mixture of chemicals depends on the genetics, parent lineage, and environmental conditions under which it was grown. This complexity is incredible and wonderful, but it's a challenge for research and accurate, reproducible medicine. Just as it would not be possible to sell a conventional medicine with more than a hundred active ingredients, it's not possible to test or regulate a whole plant medicine of that complexity. Ultimately, I suspect that limited combinations of cannabinoids in exact dose-delivery formulations will dominate the medical market. These specific products will be linked to treatment of individual symptoms and diseases based on what is certain to be an explosion of scientific cannabis research.

Patients seeking legitimate medicine will demand and expect cannabis medicines to be available through pharmacies and a safe, regulated medical marketplace. Those professional societies that currently endorse a melding of the recreational and medical streams will be proven wrong. It would not be safe, or reasonable, to expect a child with epilepsy, or an older patient with multiple sclerosis to fend for themselves in a recreational outlet in order to discover a recreational formulation that might help them. No, what these patients will have in the future is access to more refined and specific medical cannabis medication that is supported by scientific research data and prescribed by health care providers. Cannabis medicine will be treated for what it is: a remarkable natural medicine. That is the future, and here it comes.

ACKNOWLEDGEMENTS

The process of writing and publishing a book is rarely a solitary endeavour, and that was certainly the case here. I am aware that a potential hazard of writing an acknowledgements section is the difficult choice between a long and endless thank-you list and not including important people who were helpful. I hope that I am on the correct side of that choice, and I apologize to those whom I have not personally thanked.

I would like to start by thanking family and friends who supported my potentially crazy decision to leave a career in clinical surgery to pursue full-time work in the emerging field of cannabis medicine. Had that leap of faith not occurred, this book would never have been written. It is an exciting time to be part of the re-emergence of this remarkable natural medicine, and I am incredibly grateful for the opportunity.

The genesis of *Medical Cannabis in Canada* was the result of compiling answers to frequently asked questions from patients and health care providers during my lectures on medical cannabis. Therefore, a significant debt of gratitude goes to all of those people who attended the lectures and asked such good questions. Without the groundswell of support from patients, the stigma around medical cannabis wouldn't have ended.

The support needed to turn my educational content into a formal publication wouldn't have occurred without the help of my friends and colleagues at Natural Health Services. Thanks to all of them, with special thanks to Brian Vass for help in preparing an initial manuscript draft.

Once the initial content was turned into a completed draft, I required the help of professionals to get the book across the finish line. I had the pleasure of working with an excellent editor who managed to make the required process of revisions and section edits manageable and mostly fun. Thank you to my editor Andrea Maxie.

Additional thanks go to publicist Debby de Groot at MDG and Associates, distributor Rob Dawson at Georgetown Publications, and book publishing specialist Karen Milner at Milner & Associates.

Finally, I would like to thank my wife, Katharine, for agreeing to use her literature training for feedback and proofreading assistance, and my children, Henry, Charlotte, and Lily, for tolerating the many long hours where Dad was sequestered away on the computer wearing noise-cancelling headphones.

Thank you all. I could not have done this without your help.

RESOURCES

Canadian Cannabis Surveys (Health Canada)
Annual survey that captures Canadian perspectives on, and experiences with, cannabis

https://www.canada.ca/en/services/health/publications/drugs-health-products/canadian-cannabis-survey-2018-summary.html

https://www.canada.ca/en/health-canada/services/publications/drugs-health-products/canadian-cannabis-survey-2017-summary.html

Cannabis for Medical Purposes under the Cannabis Act: Information and Improvements (Health Canada)
Current information relevant to medical cannabis patients under the new Cannabis Act

https://www.canada.ca/en/health-canada/services/drugs-medication/cannabis/medical-use-cannabis.html

Cannabis in Canada (Health Canada)
Access to Health Canada's cannabis information resources

https://www.canada.ca/cannabis

Cannabis Resources (Royal College of Physicians and Surgeons of Canada)
Links to cannabis-related resources compiled by the Royal College of Physicians and Surgeons

https://ceomessage.royalcollege.ca/2018/10/16/cannabis-use-guidelines-links-to-resources/#GoC

Cannabis Resources for Family Physicians (College of Family Physicians of Canada)
Cannabis guidleines and resources aimed at primary care physicians

https://www.cfpc.ca/cannabis-resources/

Cannabis: Resources for Physicians (Doctors of British Columbia)
Cannabis guidelines and resources for practicing physicians

https://www.doctorsofbc.ca/resource-centre/
cannabis-resources-physicians

Grow-at-Home Plant Calculator (Health Canada)
Link to calculator tool for determing how many cannabis plants can be grown at home

http://www.healthycanadians.gc.ca/drugs-products-medicaments-
produits/buying-using-achat-utilisation/cannabis-medical/
access-acces/personal-production-personnelle/calculator-
calculatrice-eng.php

Information for Health Care Professionals on Cannabis (Health Canada)
Link to document prepared by Health Canada to provide information on the use of cannabis and cannabinoids for medical purposes

https://www.canada.ca/en/health-canada/services/drugs-
medication/cannabis/information-medical-practitioners/
information-health-care-professionals-cannabis-cannabinoids.html

Review of Cannabis Health Effects (National Academies)
Link to review and summary of evidence supporting the use of cannabis as medicine

http://nationalacademies.org/hmd/Reports/2017/health-effects-of-
cannabis-and-cannabinoids.aspx

GLOSSARY OF TERMS AND ABBREVIATIONS

2-AG (2-Arachidonoylglycerol) is an endocannabinoid chemical produced in our bodies that interacts with cell surface receptors to regulate numerous physiological functions.

Anandamide (N-arachidonoylethanolamine) is an endocannabinoid chemical produced in our bodies that interacts with cell surface receptors to regulate numerous physiological functions.

Antioxidants are chemicals, including some produced naturally by plants, that are able to neutralize and counter the potentially negative effects of compounds known as free radicals that are generated as the result of normal metabolism.

Blinded studies refer to scientific studies in which either the participants, investigators, or both are unaware of which substance or treatment the study subjects are receiving, in contrast to open-label studies where all parties are aware. Blinded studies may be single, double, or triple blinded. In **single-blinded** studies, the test subjects or participants are unaware which treatment they are receiving during the course of the study. In **double-blinded** studies, both the test subjects and the investigators are unaware of which treatments are being received during the course of the study. In **triple-blinded** studies, also known as fully-blinded studies, the test subjects, investigators, and data analysts/statisticians are all unaware of which group received which treatment until after results are finalized.

Breakthrough pain is sudden, severe pain that is occurring despite use of regular background pain meds. For instance, a patient on slow-release medicine may also need short-acting medicine for their breakthrough pain.

Cannabaceae is the plant family that includes cannabis, hops, and hackberries.

Cannabinoids are chemical compounds that bind to cannabinoid receptors.

Cannabinoid receptors are structures present on surface of cells that interact and/or bind with cannabinoids.

Cannabis is both the genus name of the cannabis plant and a general term used to refer to the plant and its products. When referring to the plant, the general term includes all varietals, such as indica, sativa, and hemp.

CB1 receptors are endogenous cell-surface receptors, present primarily in the central and peripheral nervous systems, that interact with both endogenous and plant cannabinoid chemicals to exert a variety of physiological effects.

CB2 receptors are endogenous cell surface receptors, present primarily in immune and peripheral organ tissues, that interact with both endogenous and plant cannabinoid chemicals to exert a variety of physiological effects.

CBD (cannabidiol) is the dominant non-psychotropic chemical produced by the cannabis plant that has extensive medicinal properties.

Cesamet is the brand name for nabilone, a synthetic form of THC.

Crossover studies are scientific studies in which test subject participants cross over from one treatment to another during the course of the trial.

Decarboxylation is the process of converting acidic cannabinoids present in the raw plant into their more biologically active forms by removing a carboxyl group, usually by using heat.

Dronabinol is a synthetic form of THC sold under the brand name Marinol.

ECS (endocannabinoid system) is a widespread neurotransmitter-like system that is comprised of cannabinoid receptors, endocannabinoid chemicals that act on those receptors, and enzymes and related chemicals that aid in the system's normal function.

Edibles are food or beverage products that have been deliberately infused with cannabis or cannabis extraction products.

Endocannabinoids are chemicals produced within our bodies that exert effects via cannabinoid receptors.

Endogenous refers to something occurring or originating naturally from within our bodies.

Entourage effect is the synergistic effect of multiple cannabis plant chemicals working together.

Epidiolex is a highly purified proprietary pharmaceutical cannabis extract that is predominantly composed of cannabidiol (CBD), recently FDA-approved for treatment of pediatric epilepsy.

G proteins (guanine nucleotide-binding proteins) are a common group of cellular proteins that often act as switches or messengers within cells.

Hash (*also* hashish) is a traditional form of concentrating cannabis by collecting and compressing cannabis resin.

High is a colloquial term that refers to the euphoria, relaxation, and potential cognitive distortion that results from cannabis intoxication.

Hyperemesis is excessive vomiting, and cannabis use has been linked to both an acute (early) and a chronic (delayed) form of hyperemesis.

Indica is a varietal of cannabis plant, originally from the Indian subcontinent, classified by Jean-Baptiste Lamarck in 1785 as *Cannabis indica*.

Joint is a colloquial term for a rolled cannabis cigarette.

LPs (licensed producers) are companies in Canada that hold the required federal licence to cultivate, process, and/or sell cannabis products for either medical or non-medical purposes.

Marijuana (*also* marihuana or mariguana) is a colloquial term for medical and recreational cannabis that is falling out of favour due to its association with racist anti-cannabis propaganda.

Marinol is the brand name for dronabinol, a synthetic form of THC.

Medical cannabis refers to products made from the cannabis plant that are manufactured and/or used specifically for the medical treatment and relief of disease and bothersome symptoms. These products are typically low in THC and higher in non-psychotropic cannabinoids, such as CBD.

Nabilone is a synthetic THC product, sold under the brand name Cesamet.

Nabiximols is a a highly purified patented pharmaceutical THC and CBD extract, sold under the brand name Sativex.

Neuromodulators are chemicals that alter or modulate the function of neurotransmitters.

Neurotransmitters are naturally produced chemical messengers in our bodies that send signals across neural junctions.

Open-label studies are studies in which both test subjects and investigators know which treatment is being administered, in contrast to blinded studies where at least one party does not know.

Pathogenesis is the mechanism or manner by which a disease progresses.

Phytocannabinoids are chemicals produced in the cannabis plant that exert effects via cannabinoid receptors.

Potentiating effects occur when the combined effects of two agents are greater than the sum of the effects of the agents alone.

Preclinical research refers to basic science studies in the lab or in animals that precede human trials.

Prospective trials are scientific studies that examine for future outcomes during the study period (as compared to retrospective studies, which look back in time for factors that influenced already established outcomes).

Psychoactive refers to a chemical substance that alters brain function, often to the point of changes in perception and cognition and possibly to the point of impairment and degradation of function. This is how the term is used in this book, but by strict definition any compound that alters central nervous system function is psychoactive, although not all psychoactive substances cause impairment.

Receptors are external cellular components that bind to and/or react with chemical messengers in order to cause cellular responses.

Recreational cannabis refers to cannabis products that are used with the intention of producing a recreational euphoriant, relaxant, or sensory stimulant experience. These products are typically high in THC.

Sativa is a varietal of the cannabis plant, classified by botanist Carl Linnaeus in 1753 as *Cannabis sativa*.

Sativex is the brand name for nabiximols, a highly purified patented pharmaceutical extract containing balanced THC and CBD.

Self-limited effects are side effects that resolve or go away on their own.

Serotonergic refers to chemicals that affect or modify the actions of the neurotransmitter serotonin in the body.

Shatter is a potent form of high-THC cannabis extract used primarily by recreational users that is translucent and fragile like plastic or glass. It can shatter into pieces and is typically heated and inhaled.

Single-arm trials are relatively simple studies where an entire single study group is given a single treatment and then followed over time to determine the results.

Synthetic cannabinoids are laboratory-manufactured chemicals that are often similar or identical in structure to individual plant cannabinoids and exert effects via cannabinoid receptors.

THC (delta9-tetrahydrocanabinol) is the dominant psychotropic chemical produced by the cannabis plant. It is the chemical that produces most of the cannabis recreational effect, and it also has extensive medicinal properties.

Upregulation refers to the body producing an increased number of cell receptors, which is often the result of a response to a corresponding change in the quantity, function, or degradation of underlying chemical messengers.

Vaporizers are mechanical devices used to heat cannabis products to the point where the cannabinoid chemicals boil and become available as vapour for inhalation.

Whole plant medicine refers to directly using parts of the whole natural cannabis plant (like the leaves or flower/bud) versus using individual extracted components (like purified CBD or THC).

ABOUT THE AUTHOR

Mark H. Kimmins, MD, FRCSC, FACS, FASCRS, is the president of Natural Health Services, a patient-centered medical cannabis clinic, and the medical director of its parent company, Sunniva. He is a medical doctor who is board certified in both the US and Canada and before entering the medical cannabis world, Mark practised as a colorectal surgeon and teaching physician for over fifteen years in Seattle, Washington, and Anchorage, Alaska.

Mark's interest in medical cannabis started with a personal belief in the benefits of this natural plant and developed further with first hand observation of the positive therapeutic effects in both patients and sick family members. His work now includes evaluating medical cannabis literature and providing evidence-based education to both physicians and patients. He looks forward to the day when the stigma around cannabis is gone, and cannabinoids are widely acknowledged as legitimate medicine.

Mark lives with his wife, three children, and multiple pets on the west coast of British Columbia, Canada.

REFERENCES

1. Pringle, H. Ice age communities may be earliest known net hunters. *Science.* **277**, 1203–1204 (1997). doi:10.1126/science.277.5330.1203

2. Fleming, M. & Clarke, R. Physical evidence for the antiquity of *Cannabis sativa* L. *Journal of the International Hemp Association* **5**, (1998).

3. Li, H.-L. An archaeological and historical account of cannabis in China. *Econ. Bot.* **28**, 437–448 (1974).

4. Touw, M. The religious and medicinal uses of Cannabis in China, India and Tibet. *J. Psychoactive Drugs* **13**, 23–34 (1981).

5. Brand, E. J. & Zhao, Z. Cannabis in Chinese medicine: are some traditional indications referenced in ancient literature related to cannabinoids? *Front. Pharmacol.* **8**, 108 (2017). doi:10.3389/fphar.2017.00108

6. Russo, E. B. History of cannabis and its preparations in saga, science, and sobriquet. *Chem. Biodivers.* **4**, 1614–1648 (2007). doi: 10.1002/cbdv.200790144

7. Butrica, J. L. The medical use of cannabis among the Greeks and Romans. *J. Cannabis Ther.* **2**, 51–70 (2002). doi:10.1300/J175v02n02_04

8. Burton, R. *The Anatomy of Melancholy.* (New York Review Books, 2001).

9. Culpeper, N. *The Complete Herbal.* (2015). Available at: http://www.gutenberg. org/files/49513/49513-h/49513-h.htm

10. Gray, S. F. *A Supplement to the Pharmacopoeia: Being a Treatise on Pharmacology in General.* (Thomas and George Underwood, 1821).

11. Moreau, J. J. *Hashish and Mental Illness.* (Raven Press, 1973).

12. O'Shaughnessy, W. B. On the preparations of the Indian hemp, or gunjah (*Cannabis indica*): their effects on the animal system in health, and their utility in the treatment of tetanus and other convulsive diseases. *Prov. Med. J. Retrosp. Med. Sci.* **5**, 363–369 (1843).

13. O'Shaughnessy, W. B. *The Bengal Pharmacopoeia, and General Conspectus of Medicinal Plants.* (Bishop's College Press, 1844).

14. Reynolds, J. R. On the therapeutical uses and toxic effects of *Cannabis indica*. *Lancet* **135**, 637–638 (1890). doi:10.1016/S0140-6736(02)18723-X

15. Indian Hemp Drugs Commission. *Report of the Indian Hemp Drug Commission, 1893-94.* (Government Central Printing Office, 1894).

16. Carstairs, C. *Jailed for Possession: Illegal Drug Use, Regulation, and Power in Canada, 1920–1961.* (University of Toronto Press, 2010).

17. Fox, S. H., Henry, B., Hill, M., Crossman, A. & Brotchie, J. Stimulation of cannabinoid receptors reduces levodopa-induced dyskinesia in the MPTP-lesioned nonhuman primate model of Parkinson's disease. *Mov. Disord.* **17**, 1180–1187 (2002). doi: 10.1002/mds.10289

18. Abel, E. L. Marijuana on trial: the Panama Canal Zone report. *Int. J. Addict.* **17**, 667–678 (1982). doi:10.3109/10826088209053010

19. Musto, D. F. The Marihuana Tax Act of 1937. *Arch. Gen. Psychiatry* **26**, 101 (1972). doi:10.1001/archpsyc.1972.01750200005002

20. Richard Nixon Foundation. *Public Enemy Number One: a Pragmatic Approach to America's Drug Problem*. (2016). Available at: https://www.nixonfoundation.org/2016/06/26404/

21. Walmsley, R. *World Prison Population List, Tenth Edition*. (2013). Available at: http://www.prisonstudies.org/sites/default/files/resources/downloads/wppl_10.pdf

22. Gasnier, L. *Reefer Madness*. (George A. Hirliman Productions, 1936).

23. Mayor's Committee on Marihuana. *The Marihuana Problem in the City of New York: Sociological, Medical, Psychological, and Pharmacological Studies*. (City of New York, 1944).

24. Commission of Inquiry into the Non-medical Use of Drugs. *Final report of the Commission of Inquiry into the Non-medical Use of Drugs*. (Health Canada, 1973).

25. United States. *Marihuana: a Signal of Misunderstanding; the Official Report of the National Commission on Marihuana and Drug Abuse*. (1972).

26. Statistics Canada. *Police-reported Crime Statistics in Canada, 2017*. (2018). Available at: https://www150.statcan.gc.ca/n1/pub/85-002-x/2018001/article/54974-eng.htm

27. American Civil Liberties Union. *Marijuana Arrests by the Numbers*. (2019). Available at: https://www.aclu.org/gallery/marijuana-arrests-numbers

28. Bonhomme, J., Stephens, T. & Braithwaite, R. African-American males in the United States prison system: impact on family and community. *J. Men's Heal. Gend.* **3**, 223–226 (2006). doi:10.1016/j.jmhg.2006.06.003

29. National Association for the Advancement of Colored People. *Criminal Justice Fact Sheet*. (2019). Available at: https://www.naacp.org/criminal-justice-fact-sheet

30. Rankin, J., Contenta, S. & Bailey, A. Toronto marijuana arrests reveal 'startling' racial divide. *Toronto Star* (2017). Available at: https://www.thestar.com/news/insight/2017/07/06/toronto-marijuana-arrests-reveal-startling-racial-divide.html

31. Washington et al v. Sessions et al, No. 1:2017cv05625 - Document 64 (S.D.N.Y. 2018) :: Justia. (2017).

32. Lehmann, J. Canadian teens lead developed world in cannabis use: UNICEF report. *Globe and Mail* (2013). Available at: https://www.theglobeandmail.com/news/national/canadian-teens-lead-developed-world-in-cannabis-use-unicef-report/article11221668/

33. Deloitte. *A Society in Transition, an Industry Ready to Bloom: 2018 Cannabis Report*. (2018). Available at: https://www2.deloitte.com/content/dam/Deloitte/ca/Documents/consulting/ca-cannabis-2018-report-en.PDF

34. Statistics Canada. *Cannabis Economic Account, Second Quarter 2018*. (2018). Available at: https://www150.statcan.gc.ca/n1/daily-quotidien/180824/dq180824e-eng.htm

35. *Canadian Charter of Rights and Freedoms*, s 7, Part I of the *Constitution Act*, 1982, being Schedule B to the *Canada Act* 1982 (UK), 1982, c 11.

36. R. v. Parker, 2000 CanLII 5762 (ON CA), 146 C.C.C. (3d) 193. (2000).

37. Grover, J. & Glasser, M. Pesticides and pot: what's california smoking? *NBCUniversal Media* (2017). Available at: https://www.nbclosangeles.com/news/local/I-Team-Marijuana-Pot-Pesticide-California-414536763.html

38. Raber, J. C., Elzinga, S. & Kaplan, C. Understanding dabs: contamination concerns of cannabis concentrates and cannabinoid transfer during the act of dabbing. *J. Toxicol. Sci.* **40**, 797–803 (2015). doi:10.2131/jts.40.797

39. Aizpurua-Olaizola, O. *et al.* Evolution of the cannabinoid and terpene content during the growth of cannabis sativa plants from different chemotypes. *J. Nat. Prod.* **79**, 324–331 (2016). doi:10.1021/acs.jnatprod.5b00949

40. Kimmins, M. H. *Trends in Canadian Medical Cannabis Clinics*. Unpublished report. (2018).

41. Devinsky, O. *et al.* Trial of cannabidiol for drug-resistant seizures in the Dravet syndrome. *N. Engl. J. Med.* **376**, 2011–2020 (2017). doi:10.1056/NEJMoa1611618

42. Russo, E. B. Taming THC: potential cannabis synergy and phytocannabinoid-terpenoid entourage effects. *Br. J. Pharmacol.* **163**, 1344–1364 (2011). doi:10.1111/j.1476-5381.2011.01238.x

43. Thompson, G. R., Fleischman, R. W., Rosenkrantz, H. & Braude, M. C. Oral and intravenous toxicity of delta9-tetrahydrocannabinol in rhesus monkeys. *Toxicol. Appl. Pharmacol.* **27**, 648–665 (1974).

44. Wang, T., Collet, J.-P., Shapiro, S. & Ware, M. A. Adverse effects of medical cannabinoids: a systematic review. *Can. Med. Assoc. J.* **178**, 1669–1678 (2008). doi:10.1503/cmaj.071178

45. Devane, W. A., Dysarz, F. A., Johnson, M. R., Melvin, L. S. & Howlett, A. C. Determination and characterization of a cannabinoid receptor in rat brain. *Mol. Pharmacol.* **34**, 605–613 (1988).

46. Munro, S., Thomas, K. L. & Abu-Shaar, M. Molecular characterization of a peripheral receptor for cannabinoids. *Nature* **365**, 61–65 (1993). doi:10.1038/365061a0

47. Russo, E. B. Clinical endocannabinoid deficiency (CECD): can this concept explain therapeutic benefits of cannabis in migraine, fibromyalgia, irritable bowel syndrome and other treatment-resistant conditions? *Neuro Endocrinol. Lett.* **25**, 31–39 (2004).

48. Sorensen, C. J., DeSanto, K., Borgelt, L., Phillips, K. T. & Monte, A. A. Cannabinoid hyperemesis syndrome: diagnosis, pathophysiology, and treatment—a systematic review. *J. Med. Toxicol.* **13**, 71–87 (2017). doi:10.1007/s13181-016-0595-z

49. Lapoint, J. *et al.* Cannabinoid hyperemesis syndrome: public health implications and a novel model treatment guideline. *West. J. Emerg. Med.* **19**, 380–386 (2018). doi:10.5811/westjem.2017.11.36368

50. Galli, J. A., Sawaya, R. A. & Friedenberg, F. K. Cannabinoid hyperemesis syndrome. *Curr. Drug Abuse Rev.* **4**, 241–249 (2011).

51. Soriano-Co, M., Batke, M. & Cappell, M. S. The cannabis hyperemesis syndrome characterized by persistent nausea and vomiting, abdominal pain, and compulsive bathing associated with chronic marijuana use: a report of eight cases in the United States. *Dig. Dis. Sci.* **55**, 3113–3119 (2010). doi:10.1007/s10620-010-1131-7

52. Pergolizzi Jr., J. V., LeQuang, J. A. & Bisney, J. F. Cannabinoid hyperemesis. *Med. Cannabis Cannabinoids* **1**, 73–95 (2018). doi:10.1159/000494992

53. Sunku, B. Cyclic vomiting syndrome: a disorder of all ages. *Gastroenterol. Hepatol.* **5**, 507–515 (2009).

54. Budney, A. J., Roffman, R., Stephens, R. S. & Walker, D. Marijuana dependence and its treatment. *Addict. Sci. Clin. Pract.* **4**, 4–16 (2007).

55. Gobbi, G. *et al.* Association of cannabis use in adolescence and risk of depression, anxiety, and suicidality in young adulthood: a systematic review and meta-analysis. *JAMA Psychiatry* (2019). doi:10.1001/jamapsychiatry.2018.4500

56. College of Family Physicians of Canada. *Authorizing Dried Cannabis for Chronic Pain or Anxiety: Preliminary Guidance from the College of Family Physicians of Canada.* (2014). Available at: https://www.cfpc.ca/uploadedfiles/resources/_pdfs/authorizing%20dried%20cannabis%20for%20chronic%20pain%20or%20anxiety.pdf

57. Health Canada. *Consumer Information—Cannabis (Marihuana, Marijuana).* (2016). Available at: https://www.canada.ca/en/health-canada/services/drugs-medication/cannabis/licensed-producers/consumer-information-cannabis.html

58. The Society of Obstetricians and Gynaecologists of Canada. *SOGC Position Statement: Marijuana Use During Pregnancy.* (2017). Available at: https://www.sogc.org/news-items/index.html?id=169

59. American College of Obstetricians and Gynecologists. *ACOG Committee Opinion: Marijuana Use During Pregnancy and Lactation.* (2017). Available at: https://www.acog.org/Clinical-Guidance-and-Publications/Committee-Opinions/Committee-on-Obstetric-Practice/Marijuana-Use-During-Pregnancy-and-Lactation?IsMobileSet=false

60. Young-Wolff, K. C. *et al.* Trends in self-reported and biochemically tested marijuana use among pregnant females in California from 2009-2016. *JAMA* **318**, 2490–2491 (2017). doi:10.1001/jama.2017.17225

61. Park, F., Potukuchi, P. K., Moradi, H. & Kovesdy, C. P. Cannabinoids and the kidney: effects in health and disease. *Am. J. Physiol. Physiol.* **313**, F1124–F1132 (2017). doi:10.1152/ajprenal.00290.2017

62. Gabbay, E., Avraham, Y., Ilan, Y., Israeli, E. & Berry, E. M. Endocannabinoids and liver disease—review. *Liver Int.* **25**, 921–926 (2005). doi:10.1111/j.1478-3231.2005.01180.x

63. Adejumo, A. C. *et al.* Cannabis use is associated with reduced prevalence of progressive stages of alcoholic liver disease. *Liver Int.* **38**, 1475–1486 (2018). doi:10.1111/liv.13696

64. Canadian Lung Association. *Cannabis Position Statement.* (2018). Available at: https://www.lung.ca/cannabis

65. American Thoracic Society. Smoking marijuana and the lungs. *Am. J. Respir. Crit. Care Med.* **195**, 5–6 (2017).

66. Penner, E. A., Buettner, H. & Mittleman, M. A. The impact of marijuana use on glucose, insulin, and insulin resistance among US adults. *Am. J. Med.* **126**, 583–589 (2013). doi:10.1016/j.amjmed.2013.03.002

67. Allan, G. M. *et al.* Systematic review of systematic reviews for medical cannabinoids: pain, nausea and vomiting, spasticity, and harms. *Can. Fam. Physician* **64**, e78–e94 (2018).

68. Centre for Evidence-Based Medicine. (2019). Available at: https://www.cebm.net/

69. Cyr, C. *et al.* Cannabis in palliative care: current challenges and practical recommendations. *Ann. Palliat. Med.* **7**, 463–477 (2018). doi:10.21037/apm.2018.06.04

70. Braun, I. M. *et al.* Medical oncologists' beliefs, practices, and knowledge regarding marijuana used therapeutically: a nationally representative survey study. *J. Clin. Oncol.* **36**, 1957–1962 (2018). doi:10.1200/JCO.2017.76.1221

71. Bar-Lev Schleider, L. *et al.* Prospective analysis of safety and efficacy of medical cannabis in large unselected population of patients with cancer. *Eur. J. Intern. Med.* **49**, 37–43 (2018). doi:10.1016/j.ejim.2018.01.023

72. National Academies of Sciences, Engineering, and Medicine. *The Health Effects of Cannabis and Cannabinoids: the Current State of Evidence and Recommendations for Research.* (2017). Available at: https://www.nap.edu/resource/24625/Cannabis_committee_conclusions.pdf

73. Stockings, E. *et al.* Cannabis and cannabinoids for the treatment of people with chronic noncancer pain conditions: a systematic review and meta-analysis of controlled and observational studies. *Pain* **159**, 1932–1954 (2018). doi:10.1097/j.pain.0000000000001293

74. Bidwell, L. C., Henry, E. A., Willcutt, E. G., Kinnear, M. K. & Ito, T. A. Childhood and current ADHD symptom dimensions are associated with more severe cannabis outcomes in college students. *Drug Alcohol Depend.* **135**, 88–94 (2014). doi:10.1016/j.drugalcdep.2013.11.013

75. Mitchell, J. T., Sweitzer, M. M., Tunno, A. M., Kollins, S. H. & McClernon, F. J. 'I use weed for my ADHD': A qualitative analysis of online forum discussions on cannabis use and ADHD. *PLoS One* **11**, e0156614 (2016). doi:10.1371/journal.pone.0156614

76. Cooper, R. *et al.* Cannabinoids in attention-deficit/hyperactivity disorder: a randomised-controlled trial. *Eur. Neuropsychopharmacol.* **27**, 795–808 (2017). doi:10.1016/j.euroneuro.2017.05.005

77. Amtmann, D., Weydt, P., Johnson, K. L., Jensen, M. P. & Carter, G. T. Survey of cannabis use in patients with amyotrophic lateral sclerosis. *Am. J. Hosp. Palliat. Med.* **21**, 95–104 (2004). doi:10.1177/104990910402100206

78. Weber, M., Goldman, B. & Truniger, S. Tetrahydrocannabinol (THC) for cramps in amyotrophic lateral sclerosis: a randomised, double-blind crossover trial. *J. Neurol. Neurosurgery, Psychiatry* **81**, 1135–1140 (2010). doi:10.1136/jnnp.2009.200642

79. Giacoppo, S. & Mazzon, E. Can cannabinoids be a potential therapeutic tool in amyotrophic lateral sclerosis? *Neural Regen. Res.* **11**, 1896–1899 (2016). doi:10.4103/1673-5374.197125

80. Carter, G. T., Abood, M. E., Aggarwal, S. K. & Weiss, M. D. Cannabis and amyotrophic lateral sclerosis: hypothetical and practical applications, and a call for clinical trials. *Am. J. Hosp. Palliat. Care* **27**, 347–356 (2010). doi:10.1177/1049909110369531

81. Campbell, V. A. & Gowran, A. Alzheimer's disease; taking the edge off with cannabinoids? *Br. J. Pharmacol.* **152**, 655–662 (2007). doi:10.1038/sj.bjp.0707446

82. Iuvone, T. *et al.* Neuroprotective effect of cannabidiol, a non-psychoactive component from Cannabis sativa, on beta-amyloid-induced toxicity in PC12 cells. *J. Neurochem.* **89**, 134–141 (2004). doi:10.1111/j.1471-4159.2003.02327.x

83. Eubanks, L. M. *et al.* A molecular link between the active component of marijuana and alzheimer's disease pathology. *Mol. Pharm.* **3**, 773–777 (2006). doi:10.1021/mp060066m

84. Cao, C. *et al.* The potential therapeutic effects of THC on Alzheimer's disease. *J. Alzheimer's Dis.* **42**, 973–984 (2014). doi:10.3233/JAD-140093

85. Shelef, A. *et al.* Safety and efficacy of medical cannabis oil for behavioral and psychological symptoms of dementia: an-open label, add-on, pilot study. *J. Alzheimer's Dis.* **51**, 15–19 (2016). doi:10.3233/JAD-150915

86. Crippa, J. A. *et al.* Cannabis and anxiety: a critical review of the evidence. *Hum. Psychopharmacol.* **24**, 515–523 (2009). doi:10.1002/hup.1048

87. Woolridge, E. *et al.* Cannabis use in HIV for pain and other medical symptoms. *J. Pain Symptom Manag.* **29**, 358–367 (2005). doi:10.1016/j.jpainsymman.2004.07.011

88. Crippa, J. A. de S. *et al.* Effects of cannabidiol (CBD) on regional cerebral blood flow. *Neuropsychopharmacology* **29**, 417–426 (2004). doi:10.1038/sj.npp.1300340

89. Bergamaschi, M. M. *et al.* Cannabidiol reduces the anxiety induced by simulated public speaking in treatment-naïve social phobia patients. *Neuropsychopharmacology* **36**, 1219–1226 (2011). doi:10.1038/npp.2011.6

90. Bhattacharyya, S. *et al.* Effect of cannabidiol on medial temporal, midbrain, and striatal dysfunction in people at clinical high risk of psychosis: a randomized clinical trial. *JAMA Psychiatry* **75**, 1107–1117 (2018). doi:10.1001/jamapsychiatry.2018.2309

91. Gui, H. *et al.* Expression of cannabinoid receptor 2 and its inhibitory effects on synovial fibroblasts in rheumatoid arthritis. *Rheumatology* **53**, 802–809 (2014). doi:10.1093/rheumatology/ket447

92. Blake, D. R., Robson, P., Ho, M., Jubb, R. W. & McCabe, C. S. Preliminary assessment of the efficacy, tolerability and safety of a cannabis-based medicine (Sativex) in the treatment of pain caused by rheumatoid arthritis. *Rheumatology* **45**, 50–52 (2006). doi:10.1093/rheumatology/kei183

93. Hammell, D. C. *et al.* Transdermal cannabidiol reduces inflammation and pain-related behaviours in a rat model of arthritis. *Eur. J. Pain* **20**, 936–948 (2016). doi:10.1002/ejp.818

94. Philpott, H. T., O'Brien, M. & McDougall, J. J. Attenuation of early phase inflammation by cannabidiol prevents pain and nerve damage in rat osteoarthritis. *Pain* **158**, 2442–2451 (2017). doi:10.1097/j.pain.0000000000001052

95. Richards, B. L., Whittle, S. L. & Buchbinder, R. Neuromodulators for pain management in rheumatoid arthritis. *Cochrane Database Syst. Rev.* **1**, CD008921 (2012). doi:10.1002/14651858.CD008921.pub2

96. Katz-Talmor, D., Katz, I., Porat-Katz, B.-S. & Shoenfeld, Y. Cannabinoids for the treatment of rheumatic diseases—where do we stand? *Nat. Rev. Rheumatol.* **14**, 488–498 (2018). doi:10.1038/s41584-018-0025-5

97. Hartley, J. P., Nogrady, S. G. & Seaton, A. Bronchodilator effect of delta1-tetrahydrocannabinol. *Br. J. Clin. Pharmacol.* **5**, 523–525 (1978).

98. Tashkin, D. P., Shapiro, B. J., Lee, Y. E. & Harper, C. E. Effects of smoked marijuana in experimentally induced asthma. *Am. Rev. Respir. Dis.* **112**, 377–386 (1975). doi:10.1164/arrd.1975.112.3.377

99. Pletcher, M. J. *et al.* Association between marijuana exposure and pulmonary function over 20 years. *JAMA* **307**, 173–181 (2012). doi:10.1001/jama.2011.1961

100. Hanson, A. C. & Hagerman, R. J. Serotonin dysregulation in Fragile X Syndrome: implications for treatment. *Intractable Rare Dis. Res.* **3**, 110–117 (2014). doi:10.5582/irdr.2014.01027

101. Krueger, D. D. & Brose, N. Evidence for a common endocannabinoid-related pathomechanism in autism spectrum disorders. *Neuron* **78**, 408–410 (2013). doi:10.1016/j.neuron.2013.04.030

102. Rocha, F. C. M., Dos Santos Júnior, J. G., Stefano, S. C. & da Silveira, D. X. Systematic review of the literature on clinical and experimental trials on the antitumor effects of cannabinoids in gliomas. *J. Neurooncol.* **116**, 11–24 (2014). doi:10.1007/s11060-013-1277-1

103. De Petrocellis, L. *et al.* The endogenous cannabinoid anandamide inhibits human breast cancer cell proliferation. *Proc. Natl. Acad. Sci. U. S. A.* **95**, 8375–8380 (1998).

104. Takeda, S. *et al.* Cannabidiolic acid, a major cannabinoid in fiber-type cannabis, is an inhibitor of MDA-MB-231 breast cancer cell migration. *Toxicol. Lett.* **214**, 314–319 (2012). doi:10.1016/j.toxlet.2012.08.029

105. Guzmán, M. *et al.* A pilot clinical study of delta9-tetrahydrocannabinol in patients with recurrent glioblastoma multiforme. *Br. J. Cancer* **95**, 197–203 (2006). doi:10.1038/sj.bjc.6603236

106. Marcu, J. P. *et al.* Cannabidiol enhances the inhibitory effects of delta9-tetrahydrocannabinol on human glioblastoma cell proliferation and survival. *Mol. Cancer Ther.* **9**, 180–189 (2010). doi:10.1158/1535-7163.MCT-09-0407

107. Musty, R. E. & Rossi, R. Effects of smoked cannabis and oral Δ9-tetrahydrocannabinol on nausea and emesis after cancer chemotherapy. *J. Cannabis Ther.* **1**, 29–56 (2001). doi:10.1300/J175v01n01_03

108. Tramèr, M. R. *et al.* Cannabinoids for control of chemotherapy induced nausea and vomiting: quantitative systematic review. *Br. Med. J.* **323**, 16–21 (2001).

109. Machado Rocha, F. C., Stéfano, S. C., De Cássia Haiek, R., Rosa Oliveira, L. M. Q. & Da Silveira, D. X. Therapeutic use of Cannabis sativa on chemotherapy-induced nausea and vomiting among cancer patients: systematic review and meta-analysis. *Eur. J. Cancer Care (Engl).* **17**, 431–443 (2008). doi:10.1111/j.1365-2354.2008.00917.x

110. Smith, L. A., Azariah, F., Lavender, V. T., Stoner, N. S. & Bettiol, S. Cannabinoids for nausea and vomiting in adults with cancer receiving chemotherapy. *Cochrane Database Syst. Rev.* CD009464 (2015). doi:10.1002/14651858.CD009464.pub2

111. Whiting, P. F. *et al.* Cannabinoids for medical use: a systematic review and meta-analysis. *JAMA* **313**, 2456–2473 (2015). doi:10.1001/jama.2015.6358

112. Hampson, A. J., Grimaldi, M., Axelrod, J. & Wink, D. Cannabidiol and (-)delta9-tetrahydrocannabinol are neuroprotective antioxidants. *Proc. Natl. Acad. Sci. U. S. A.* **95**, 8268–8273 (1998).

113. Hampson, A. J. *et al.* Neuroprotective antioxidants from marijuana. *Ann. N. Y. Acad. Sci.* **899**, 274–282 (2000).

114. Mori, M. A. *et al.* Cannabidiol reduces neuroinflammation and promotes neuroplasticity and functional recovery after brain ischemia. *Prog. Neuropsychopharmacol. Biol. Psychiatry* **75**, 94–105 (2017). doi:10.1016/j.pnpbp.2016.11.005

115. Weiss, L. *et al.* Cannabidiol lowers incidence of diabetes in non-obese diabetic mice. *Autoimmunity* **39**, 143–151 (2006). doi:10.1080/08916930500356674

116. Smit, E. & Crespo, C. J. Dietary intake and nutritional status of US adult marijuana users: results from the Third National Health and Nutrition Examination Survey. *Public Health Nutr.* **4**, 781–786 (2001).

117. Rajavashisth, T. B. *et al.* Decreased prevalence of diabetes in marijuana users: cross-sectional data from the National Health and Nutrition Examination Survey (NHANES) III. *Br. Med. J. Open* **2**, e000494 (2012). doi:10.1136/bmjopen-2011-000494

118. Jadoon, K. A. *et al.* Efficacy and safety of cannabidiol and tetrahydrocannabivarin on glycemic and lipid parameters in patients with type 2 diabetes: a randomized, double-blind, placebo-controlled, parallel group pilot study. *Diabetes Care* **39**, 1777–1786 (2016). doi:10.2337/dc16-0650

119. Bambico, F. R., Katz, N., Debonnel, G. & Gobbi, G. Cannabinoids elicit antidepressant-like behavior and activate serotonergic neurons through the medial prefrontal cortex. *J. Neurosci.* **27**, 11700–11711 (2007). doi:10.1523/JNEUROSCI.1636-07.2007

120. Sales, A. J., Crestani, C. C., Guimarães, F. S. & Joca, S. R. L. Antidepressant-like effect induced by cannabidiol is dependent on brain serotonin levels. *Prog. Neuropsychopharmacol. Biol. Psychiatry* **86**, 255–261 (2018). doi:10.1016/j.pnpbp.2018.06.002

121. Morrish, A. C., Hill, M. N., Riebe, C. J. N. & Gorzalka, B. B. Protracted cannabinoid administration elicits antidepressant behavioral responses in rats: role of gender and noradrenergic transmission. *Physiol. Behav.* **98**, 118–124 (2009). doi:10.1016/j.physbeh.2009.04.023

122. Bambico, F. R., Duranti, A., Nobrega, J. N. & Gobbi, G. The fatty acid amide hydrolase inhibitor URB597 modulates serotonin-dependent emotional behaviour, and serotonin1A and serotonin2A/C activity in the hippocampus. *Eur. Neuropsychopharmacol.* **26**, 578–590 (2016). doi:10.1016/j.euroneuro.2015.12.027

123. Gordon, E. & Devinsky, O. Alcohol and marijuana: effects on epilepsy and use by patients with epilepsy. *Epilepsia* **42**, 1266–1272 (2001).

124. Tzadok, M. *et al.* CBD-enriched medical cannabis for intractable pediatric epilepsy: the current Israeli experience. *Seizure* **35**, 41–44 (2016). doi:10.1016/j.seizure.2016.01.004

125. Berkovic, S. F. Cannabinoids for epilepsy—real data, at last. *N. Engl. J. Med.* **376**, 2075–2076 (2017). doi:10.1056/NEJMe1702205

126. Fitzcharles, M.-A. *et al.* 2012 Canadian guidelines for the diagnosis and management of fibromyalgia syndrome: executive summary. *Pain Res. Manag.* **18**, 119–126 (2012).

127. Schley, M. *et al.* Delta-9-THC based monotherapy in fibromyalgia patients on experimentally induced pain, axon reflex flare, and pain relief. *Curr. Med. Res. Opin.* **22**, 1269–76 (2006). doi:10.1185/030079906X112651

128. Weber, J. *et al.* Tetrahydrocannabinol (delta 9-THC) treatment in chronic central neuropathic pain and fibromyalgia patients: results of a multicenter survey. *Anesthesiol. Res. Pract.* **2009**, 1–9 (2009). doi:10.1155/2009/827290

129. Fiz, J., Durán, M., Capellà, D., Carbonell, J. & Farré, M. Cannabis use in patients with fibromyalgia: effect on symptoms relief and health-related quality of life. *PLoS One* **6**, e18440 (2011). doi:10.1371/journal.pone.0018440

130. Walitt, B., Klose, P., Fitzcharles, M.-A., Phillips, T. & Häuser, W. Cannabinoids for fibromyalgia. *Cochrane Database Syst. Rev.* **7**, CD011694 (2016). doi:10.1002/14651858.CD011694.pub2

131. Donvito, G. *et al.* The endogenous cannabinoid system: a budding source of targets for treating inflammatory and neuropathic pain. *Neuropsychopharmacology* **43**, 52–79 (2018). doi:10.1038/npp.2017.204

132. Habib, G. & Artul, S. Medical cannabis for the treatment of fibromyalgia. *J. Clin. Rheumatol. Pract. Reports Rheum. Musculoskelet. Dis.* **24**, 255–258 (2018). doi:10.1097/RHU.0000000000000702

133. Izzo, A. A. & Sharkey, K. A. Cannabinoids and the gut: new developments and emerging concepts. *Pharmacol. Ther.* **126**, 21–38 (2010). doi:10.1016/j. pharmthera.2009.12.005

134. Aviello, G., Romano, B. & Izzo, A. A. Cannabinoids and gastrointestinal motility: animal and human studies. *Eur. Rev. Med. Pharmacol. Sci.* **12 Suppl 1**, 81–93 (2008).

135. Hornby, P. J. & Prouty, S. M. Involvement of cannabinoid receptors in gut motility and visceral perception. *Br. J. Pharmacol.* **141**, 1335–1345 (2004). doi:10.1038/sj.bjp.0705783

136. Novack, G. D. Cannabinoids for treatment of glaucoma. *Curr. Opin. Ophthalmol.* **27**, 146–150 (2016). doi:10.1097/ICU.0000000000000242

137. Schwitzer, T., Schwan, R., Angioi-Duprez, K., Giersch, A. & Laprevote, V. The endocannabinoid system in the retina: from physiology to practical and therapeutic applications. *Neural Plast.* **2016**, 2916732 (2016). doi:10.1155/2016/2916732

138. Caldwell, M. The Pharmacology of Cannabinoids and Cannabimimetic Ligands in the Eye and Their Effects on Intraocular Pressure. M.Sc. thesis. (Dalhousie University, 2015).

139. Merritt, J. C., Crawford, W. J., Alexander, P. C., Anduze, A. L. & Gelbart, S. S. Effect of marihuana on intraocular and blood pressure in glaucoma. *Ophthalmology* **87**, 222–228 (1980).

140. Health Canada. *Information for Health Care Professionals: Cannabis (Marihuana, Marijuana) and the Cannabinoids.* (2018). Available at: https://www.canada.ca/en/health-canada/services/drugs-medication/cannabis/information-medical-practitioners/information-health-care-professionals-cannabis-cannabinoids.html

141. Parfieniuk, A. & Flisiak, R. Role of cannabinoids in chronic liver diseases. *World J. Gastroenterol.* **14**, 6109–6114 (2008).

142. Mallat, A., Teixeira-Clerc, F., Deveaux, V., Manin, S. & Lotersztajn, S. The endocannabinoid system as a key mediator during liver diseases: new insights and therapeutic openings. *Br. J. Pharmacol.* **163**, 1432–1440 (2011). doi:10.1111/j.1476-5381.2011.01397.x

143. Patsenker, E. & Stickel, F. Cannabinoids in liver diseases. *Clin. Liver Dis.* **7**, 21–25 (2016). doi:10.1002/cld.527

144. Hézode, C. *et al.* Daily cannabis smoking as a risk factor for progression of fibrosis in chronic hepatitis C. *Hepatology* **42**, 63–71 (2005). doi:10.1002/hep.20733

145. Sylvestre, D. L., Clements, B. J. & Malibu, Y. Cannabis use improves retention and virological outcomes in patients treated for hepatitis C. *Eur. J. Gastroenterol. Hepatol.* **18**, 1057–1063 (2006). doi:10.1097/01.meg.0000216934.22114.51

146. Pazos, M. R., Sagredo, O. & Fernández-Ruiz, J. The endocannabinoid system in Huntington's disease. *Curr. Pharm. Des.* **14**, 2317–2325 (2008).

147. Fernández-Ruiz, J., Pazos, M. R., García-Arencibia, M., Sagredo, O. & Ramos, J. A. Role of CB2 receptors in neuroprotective effects of cannabinoids. *Mol. Cell. Endocrinol.* **286**, S91–S96 (2008). doi:10.1016/j.mce.2008.01.001

148. Lastres-Becker, I. *et al.* Alleviation of motor hyperactivity and neurochemical deficits by endocannabinoid uptake inhibition in a rat model of Huntington's disease. *Synapse* **44**, 23–35 (2002). doi:10.1002/syn.10054

149. López-Sendón Moreno, J. L. *et al.* A double-blind, randomized, cross-over, placebo-controlled, pilot trial with Sativex in Huntington's disease. *J. Neurol.* **263**, 1390–1400 (2016). doi:10.1007/s00415-016-8145-9

150. Mattes, R. D., Engelman, K., Shaw, L. M. & Elsohly, M. A. Cannabinoids and appetite stimulation. *Pharmacol. Biochem. Behav.* **49**, 187–195 (1994).

151. Beal, J. E. *et al.* Long-term efficacy and safety of dronabinol for acquired immunodeficiency syndrome-associated anorexia. *J. Pain Symptom Manag.* **14**, 7–14 (1997). doi:10.1016/S0885-3924(97)00038-9

152. Haney, M., Rabkin, J., Gunderson, E. & Foltin, R. W. Dronabinol and marijuana in HIV(+) marijuana smokers: acute effects on caloric intake and mood. *Psychopharmacology (Berl).* **181**, 170–178 (2005). doi:10.1007/s00213-005-2242-2

153. Haney, M. *et al.* Dronabinol and marijuana in HIV-positive marijuana smokers: caloric intake, mood, and sleep. *J. Acquir. Immune Defic. Syndr.* **45**, 545–554 (2007). doi:10.1097/QAI.0b013e31811ed205

154. Sansone, R. A. & Sansone, L. A. Marijuana and body weight. *Innov. Clin. Neurosci.* **11**, 50–54 (2014).

155. Nagarkatti, P., Pandey, R., Rieder, S. A., Hegde, V. L. & Nagarkatti, M. Cannabinoids as novel anti-inflammatory drugs. *Future Med. Chem.* **1**, 1333–1349 (2009). doi:10.4155/fmc.09.93

156. Zurier, R. B. Prospects for cannabinoids as anti-inflammatory agents. *J. Cell. Biochem.* **88**, 462–466 (2003). doi:10.1002/jcb.10291

157. Klein, T. W. Cannabinoid-based drugs as anti-inflammatory therapeutics. *Nat. Rev. Immunol.* **5**, 400–411 (2005). doi:10.1038/nri1602

158. Liu, W. M., Fowler, D. W. & Dalgleish, A. G. Cannabis-derived substances in cancer therapy—an emerging anti-inflammatory role for the cannabinoids. *Curr. Clin. Pharmacol.* **5**, 281–287 (2010).

159. Yang, X. *et al.* Histone modifications are associated with Δ9-tetrahydrocannabinol-mediated alterations in antigen-specific T cell responses. *J. Biol. Chem.* **289**, 18707–18718 (2014). doi:10.1074/jbc.M113.545210

160. Kozela, E. *et al.* Pathways and gene networks mediating the regulatory effects of cannabidiol, a nonpsychoactive cannabinoid, in autoimmune T cells. *J. Neuroinflammation* **13**, 136 (2016). doi:10.1186/s12974-016-0603-x

161. Di Sabatino, A. *et al.* The endogenous cannabinoid system in the gut of patients with inflammatory bowel disease. *Mucosal Immunol.* **4**, 574–583 (2011). doi:10.1038/mi.2011.18

162. DiPatrizio, N. V. Endocannabinoids in the gut. *Cannabis Cannabinoid Res.* **1**, 67–77 (2016). doi:10.1089/can.2016.0001

163. Naftali, T. *et al.* Treatment of Crohn's disease with cannabis: an observational study. *Isr. Med. Assoc. J.* **13**, 455–458 (2011).

164. Lahat, A., Lang, A. & Ben-Horin, S. Impact of cannabis treatment on the quality of life, weight and clinical disease activity in inflammatory bowel disease patients: a pilot prospective study. *Digestion* **85**, 1–8 (2012). doi:10.1159/000332079

165. Naftali, T. *et al.* Cannabis induces a clinical response in patients with Crohn's disease: a prospective placebo-controlled study. *Clin. Gastroenterol. Hepatol.* **11**, 1276–1280.e1 (2013). doi:10.1016/j.cgh.2013.04.034

166. Storr, M., Devlin, S., Kaplan, G. G., Panaccione, R. & Andrews, C. N. Cannabis use provides symptom relief in patients with inflammatory bowel disease but is associated with worse disease prognosis in patients with Crohn's disease. *Inflamm. Bowel Dis.* **20**, 472–480 (2014). doi:10.1097/01.MIB.0000440982.79036. d6

167. Wong, B. S. *et al.* Pharmacogenetic trial of a cannabinoid agonist shows reduced fasting colonic motility in patients with nonconstipated irritable bowel syndrome. *Gastroenterology* **141**, 1638-1647.e1–7 (2011). doi:10.1053/j. gastro.2011.07.036

168. Camilleri, M. *et al.* Cannabinoid receptor 1 gene and irritable bowel syndrome: phenotype and quantitative traits. *Am. J. Physiol. Liver Physiol.* **304**, G553–G560 (2013). doi:10.1152/ajpgi.00376.2012

169. Volz, M. S., Siegmund, B. & Häuser, W. Efficacy, tolerability, and safety of cannabinoids in gastroenterology: a systematic review. *Schmerz* **30**, 37–46 (2016). doi:10.1007/s00482-015-0087-0

170. Russo, E. Cannabis for migraine treatment: the once and future prescription? An historical and scientific review. *Pain* **76**, 3–8 (1998).

171. Lochte, B. C., Beletsky, A., Samuel, N. K. & Grant, I. The use of cannabis for headache disorders. *Cannabis Cannabinoid Res.* **2**, 61–71 (2017). doi:10.1089/ can.2016.0033

172. Van der Schueren, B. J., Van Laere, K., Gérard, N., Bormans, G. & De Hoon, J. N. Interictal type 1 cannabinoid receptor binding is increased in female migraine patients. *Headache J. Head Face Pain* **52**, 433–440 (2012). doi:10.1111/j.1526-4610.2011.02030.x

173. Rhyne, D. N., Anderson, S. L., Gedde, M. & Borgelt, L. M. Effects of medical marijuana on migraine headache frequency in an adult population. *Pharmacotherapy* **36**, 505–510 (2016). doi:10.1002/phar.1673

174. Chong, M. S. *et al.* Cannabis use in patients with multiple sclerosis. *Mult. Scler.* **12**, 646–651 (2006). doi:10.1177/1352458506070947

175. Zajicek, J. *et al.* Cannabinoids for treatment of spasticity and other symptoms related to multiple sclerosis (CAMS study): multicentre randomised placebo-controlled trial. *Lancet* **362**, 1517–1526 (2003). doi:10.1016/ S0140-6736(03)14738-1

176. Rog, D. J., Nurmikko, T. J., Friede, T. & Young, C. A. Randomized, controlled trial of cannabis-based medicine in central pain in multiple sclerosis. *Neurology* **65**, 812–819 (2005). doi:10.1212/01.wnl.0000176753.45410.8b

177. Collin, C., Davies, P., Mutiboko, I. K., Ratcliffe, S. & Sativex Spasticity in MS Study Group. Randomized controlled trial of cannabis-based medicine in spasticity caused by multiple sclerosis. *Eur. J. Neurol.* **14**, 290–296 (2007). doi:10.1111/j.1468-1331.2006.01639.x

178. Vaney, C. *et al.* Efficacy, safety and tolerability of an orally administered cannabis extract in the treatment of spasticity in patients with multiple sclerosis: a randomized, double-blind, placebo-controlled, crossover study. *Mult. Scler.* **10**, 417–424 (2004). doi:10.1191/1352458504ms1048oa

179. Collin, C. *et al.* A double-blind, randomized, placebo-controlled, parallel-group study of Sativex, in subjects with symptoms of spasticity due to multiple sclerosis. *Neurol. Res.* **32**, 451–459 (2010). doi:10.1179/01616410 9X12590518685660

180. Svendsen, K. B., Jensen, T. S. & Bach, F. W. Does the cannabinoid dronabinol reduce central pain in multiple sclerosis? Randomised double blind placebo controlled crossover trial. *Br. Med. J.* **329**, 253–260 (2004). doi:10.1136/ bmj.38149.566979.AE

181. Corey-Bloom, J. *et al.* Smoked cannabis for spasticity in multiple sclerosis: a randomized, placebo-controlled trial. *Can. Med. Assoc. J.* **184**, 1143–1150 (2012). doi:10.1503/cmaj.110837

182. Novotna, A. *et al.* A randomized, double-blind, placebo-controlled, parallel-group, enriched-design study of nabiximols (Sativex), as add-on therapy, in subjects with refractory spasticity caused by multiple sclerosis. *Eur. J. Neurol.* **18**, 1122–1131 (2011). doi:10.1111/j.1468-1331.2010.03328.x

183. Zajicek, J. P. *et al.* Multiple sclerosis and extract of cannabis: results of the MUSEC trial. *J. Neurol. Neurosurgery, Psychiatry* **83**, 1125–1132 (2012). doi:10.1136/jnnp-2012-302468

184. Malfitano, A. M., Proto, M. C. & Bifulco, M. Cannabinoids in the management of spasticity associated with multiple sclerosis. *Neuropsychiatr. Dis. Treat.* **4**, 847–853 (2008).

185. Zajicek, J. *et al.* Effect of dronabinol on progression in progressive multiple sclerosis (CUPID): a randomised, placebo-controlled trial. *Lancet Neurol.* **12**, 857–865 (2013). doi:10.1016/S1474-4422(13)70159-5

186. Prud'homme, M., Cata, R. & Jutras-Aswad, D. Cannabidiol as an intervention for addictive behaviors: a systematic review of the evidence. *Subst. Abus. Res. Treat.* **9**, SART.S25081 (2015). doi:10.4137/SART.S25081

187. Reiman, A., Welty, M. & Solomon, P. Cannabis as a substitute for opioid-based pain medication: patient self-report. *Cannabis Cannabinoid Res.* **2**, 160–166 (2017). doi:10.1089/can.2017.0012

188. Lucas, P. Rationale for cannabis-based interventions in the opioid overdose crisis. *Harm Reduct. J.* **14**, 58 (2017). doi:10.1186/s12954-017-0183-9

189. Lucas, P. & Walsh, Z. Medical cannabis access, use, and substitution for prescription opioids and other substances: a survey of authorized medical cannabis patients. *Int. J. Drug Policy* **42**, 30–35 (2017). doi:10.1016/j.drugpo.2017.01.011

190. Lucas, P. Cannabis as an adjunct to or substitute for opiates in the treatment of chronic pain. *J. Psychoactive Drugs* **44**, 125–133 (2012). doi:10.1080/02791072.2012.684624

191. US Institute of Medicine Committee on Advancing Pain Research, Care, and Education. *Relieving Pain in America: a Blueprint for Transforming Prevention, Care, Education, and Research.* (National Academies Press, 2011). doi:10.17226/13172

192. Johnson, J. R. *et al.* Multicenter, double-blind, randomized, placebo-controlled, parallel-group study of the efficacy, safety, and tolerability of THC:CBD extract and THC extract in patients with intractable cancer-related pain. *J. Pain Symptom Manag.* **39**, 167–179 (2010). doi:10.1016/j.jpainsymman.2009.06.008

193. Abrams, D. I., Couey, P., Shade, S. B., Kelly, M. E. & Benowitz, N. L. Cannabinoid-opioid interaction in chronic pain. *Clin. Pharmacol. Ther.* **90**, 844–851 (2011). doi:10.1038/clpt.2011.188

194. Lichtman, A. H. *et al.* Results of a double-blind, randomized, placebo-controlled study of nabiximols oromucosal spray as an adjunctive therapy in advanced cancer patients with chronic uncontrolled pain. *J. Pain Symptom Manag.* **55**, 179–188.e1 (2018).

195. Blake, A. *et al.* A selective review of medical cannabis in cancer pain management. *Ann. Palliat. Med.* **6**, S215–S222 (2017). doi:10.1016/j.jpainsymman.2017.09.001

196. Ware, M. A. *et al.* Smoked cannabis for chronic neuropathic pain: a randomized controlled trial. *Can. Med. Assoc. J.* **182**, E694-701 (2010). doi:10.1503/cmaj.091414

197. Boehnke, K. F., Litinas, E. & Clauw, D. J. Medical cannabis use is associated with decreased opiate medication use in a retrospective cross-sectional survey of patients with chronic pain. *J. Pain* **17**, 739–744 (2016). doi:10.1016/j.jpain.2016.03.002

198. Bradford, A. C. & Bradford, W. D. Medical marijuana laws reduce prescription medication use in Medicare Part D. *Health Aff.* **35**, 1230–1236 (2016). doi:10.1377/hlthaff.2015.1661

199. Bruce, D., Brady, J. P., Foster, E. & Shattell, M. Preferences for medical marijuana over prescription medications among persons living with chronic conditions: alternative, complementary, and tapering uses. *J. Altern. Complement. Med.* **24**, 146–153 (2018). doi:10.1089/acm.2017.0184

200. Martín-Sánchez, E., Furukawa, T. A., Taylor, J. & Martin, J. L. R. Systematic review and meta-analysis of cannabis treatment for chronic pain. *Pain Med.* **10**, 1353–1368 (2009). doi:10.1111/j.1526-4637.2009.00703.x

201. De Gregorio, D. *et al.* Cannabidiol modulates serotonergic transmission and reverses both allodynia and anxiety-like behavior in a model of neuropathic pain. *Pain* **160**, 136–150 (2019). doi:10.1097/j.pain.0000000000001386

202. Wallace, M. *et al.* Dose-dependent effects of smoked cannabis on capsaicin-induced pain and hyperalgesia in healthy volunteers. *Anesthesiology* **107**, 785–796 (2007). doi:10.1097/01.anes.0000286986.92475.b7

203. Portenoy, R. K. *et al.* Nabiximols for opioid-treated cancer patients with poorly-controlled chronic pain: a randomized, placebo-controlled, graded-dose trial. *J. Pain* **13**, 438–449 (2012). doi:10.1016/j.jpain.2012.01.003

204. Sohler, N. L. *et al.* Cannabis use is associated with lower odds of prescription opioid analgesic use among HIV-infected individuals with chronic pain. *Subst. Use Misuse* **53**, 1602–1607 (2018). doi:10.1080/10826084.2017.1416408

205. Allan, G. M. *et al.* Simplified guideline for prescribing medical cannabinoids in primary care. *Can. Fam. Physician* **64**, 111–120 (2018).

206. Green, A. J. & De-Vries, K. Cannabis use in palliative care—an examination of the evidence and the implications for nurses. *J. Clin. Nurs.* **19**, 2454–2462 (2010). doi:10.1111/j.1365-2702.2010.03274.x

207. Fernández-Ruiz, J. The endocannabinoid system as a target for the treatment of motor dysfunction. *Br. J. Pharmacol.* **156**, 1029–1040 (2009). doi:10.1111/j.1476-5381.2008.00088.x

208. Chagas, M. H. N. *et al.* Effects of cannabidiol in the treatment of patients with Parkinson's disease: an exploratory double-blind trial. *J. Psychopharmacol.* **28**, 1088–1098 (2014). doi:10.1177/0269881114550355

209. Kindred, J. H. *et al.* Cannabis use in people with Parkinson's disease and multiple sclerosis: a web-based investigation. *Complement. Ther. Med.* **33**, 99–104 (2017). doi:10.1016/j.ctim.2017.07.002

210. Balash, Y. *et al.* Medical cannabis in Parkinson disease: real-life patients' experience. *Clin. Neuropharmacol.* **40**, 268–272 (2017). doi:10.1097/WNF.0000000000000246

211. Stampanoni Bassi, M., Sancesario, A., Morace, R., Centonze, D. & Iezzi, E. Cannabinoids in Parkinson's disease. *Cannabis Cannabinoid Res.* **2**, 21–29 (2017). doi:10.1089/can.2017.0002

212. Van Til, L. *et al. Well-being of Canadian Regular Force Veterans, Findings from LASS 2016 Survey.* (Veterans Affairs Canada, 2017). Available at: http://publications.gc.ca/collections/collection_2017/acc-vac/V32-340-2017-eng.pdf

213. Office of Mental Health and Suicide Prevention. *Suicide Among Veterans and Other Americans 2001-2014.* (Veterans Affairs Canada, 2016). Available at: https://www.mentalhealth.va.gov/docs/2016suicidedatareport.pdf

214. Dückers, M. L. A., Alisic, E. & Brewin, C. R. A vulnerability paradox in the cross-national prevalence of post-traumatic stress disorder. *Br. J. Psychiatry* **209**, 300–305 (2016). doi:10.1192/bjp.bp.115.176628

215. Bitencourt, R. M. & Takahashi, R. N. Cannabidiol as a therapeutic alternative for post-traumatic stress disorder: from bench research to confirmation in human trials. *Front. Neurosci.* **12**, 502 (2018). doi:10.3389/fnins.2018.00502

216. Greer, G. R., Grob, C. S. & Halberstadt, A. L. PTSD symptom reports of patients evaluated for the New Mexico Medical Cannabis Program. *J. Psychoactive Drugs* **46**, 73–77 (2014). doi:10.1080/02791072.2013.873843

217. Roitman, P., Mechoulam, R., Cooper-Kazaz, R. & Shalev, A. Preliminary, open-label, pilot study of add-on oral Δ9-tetrahydrocannabinol in chronic post-traumatic stress disorder. *Clin. Drug Investig.* **34**, 587–591 (2014). doi:10.1007/s40261-014-0212-3

218. Sterniczuk, R. & Whelan, J. Cannabis use among Canadian Armed Forces Veterans. *J. Mil. Veteran Fam. Heal.* **2**, 43–52 (2016). doi:10.3138/jmvfh.3836

219. Davis, A. K., Lin, L. A., Ilgen, M. A. & Bohnert, K. M. Recent cannabis use among Veterans in the United States: results from a national sample. *Addict. Behav.* **76**, 223–228 (2018). doi:10.1016/j.addbeh.2017.08.010

220. Bonn-Miller, M. O., Babson, K. A. & Vandrey, R. Using cannabis to help you sleep: heightened frequency of medical cannabis use among those with PTSD. *Drug Alcohol Depend.* **136**, 162–165 (2014). doi:10.1016/j.drugalcdep.2013.12.008

221. Walsh, Z. *et al.* Medical cannabis and mental health: a guided systematic review. *Clin. Psychol. Rev.* **51**, 15–29 (2017). doi:10.1016/j.cpr.2016.10.002

222. Segal-Gavish, H. *et al.* BDNF overexpression prevents cognitive deficit elicited by adolescent cannabis exposure and host susceptibility interaction. *Hum. Mol. Genet.* **26**, 2462–2471 (2017). doi:10.1093/hmg/ddx139

223. Hall, W. & Degenhardt, L. Cannabis use and the risk of developing a psychotic disorder. *World Psychiatry* **7**, 68–71 (2008).

224. Power, R. A. *et al.* Genetic predisposition to schizophrenia associated with increased use of cannabis. *Mol. Psychiatry* **19**, 1201–1204 (2014). doi:10.1038/mp.2014.51

225. Leweke, F. M. *et al.* Cannabidiol enhances anandamide signaling and alleviates psychotic symptoms of schizophrenia. *Transl. Psychiatry* **2**, e94–e94 (2012). doi:10.1038/tp.2012.15

226. Bíró, T., Tóth, B. I., Haskó, G., Paus, R. & Pacher, P. The endocannabinoid system of the skin in health and disease: novel perspectives and therapeutic opportunities. *Trends Pharmacol. Sci.* **30**, 411–420 (2009). doi:10.1016/j.tips.2009.05.004

227. Kupczyk, P., Reich, A. & Szepietowski, J. C. Cannabinoid system in the skin—a possible target for future therapies in dermatology. *Exp. Dermatol.* **18**, 669–679 (2009). doi:10.1111/j.1600-0625.2009.00923.x

228. Yesilyurt, O. *et al.* Topical cannabinoid enhances topical morphine antinociception. *Pain* **105**, 303–308 (2003).

229. Wilkinson, J. D. & Williamson, E. M. Cannabinoids inhibit human keratinocyte proliferation through a non-CB1/CB2 mechanism and have a potential therapeutic value in the treatment of psoriasis. *J. Dermatol. Sci.* **45**, 87–92 (2007). doi:10.1016/j.jdermsci.2006.10.009

230. Oláh, A. *et al.* Cannabidiol exerts sebostatic and antiinflammatory effects on human sebocytes. *J. Clin. Invest.* **124**, 3713–3724 (2014). doi:10.1172/JCI64628

231. Oláh, A. *et al.* Differential effectiveness of selected non-psychotropic phytocannabinoids on human sebocyte functions implicates their introduction in dry/seborrhoeic skin and acne treatment. *Exp. Dermatol.* **25**, 701–707 (2016). doi:10.1111/exd.13042

232. Babson, K. A., Sottile, J. & Morabito, D. Cannabis, cannabinoids, and sleep: a review of the literature. *Curr. Psychiatry Rep.* **19**, 23 (2017). doi:10.1007/s11920-017-0775-9

233. Cousens, K. & DiMascio, A. Delta 9 THC as an hypnotic: an experimental study of three dose levels. *Psychopharmacologia* **33**, 355–364 (1973).

234. Freemon, F. R. The effect of chronically administered delta-9-tetrahydrocannabinol upon the polygraphically monitored sleep of normal volunteers. *Drug Alcohol Depend.* **10**, 345–353 (1982).

235. Carlini, E. A. & Cunha, J. M. Hypnotic and antiepileptic effects of cannabidiol. *J. Clin. Pharmacol.* **21**, 417S–427S (1981).

236. Ware, M. A., Fitzcharles, M.-A., Joseph, L. & Shir, Y. The effects of nabilone on sleep in fibromyalgia: results of a randomized controlled trial. *Anesth. Analg.* **110**, 604–610 (2010). doi:10.1213/ANE.0b013e3181c76f70

237. Carley, D. W. *et al.* Pharmacotherapy of apnea by cannabimimetic enhancement, the PACE clinical trial: effects of dronabinol in obstructive sleep apnea. *Sleep* **41**, zsx184 (2018). doi:10.1093/sleep/zsx184

238. Drossel, C., Forchheimer, M. & Meade, M. A. Characteristics of individuals with spinal cord injury who use cannabis for therapeutic purposes. *Top. Spinal Cord Inj. Rehabil.* **22**, 3–12 (2016). doi:10.1310/sci2201-3

239. Dunn, M. & Davis, R. The perceived effects of marijuana on spinal cord injured males. *Paraplegia* **12**, 175 (1974). doi:10.1038/sc.1974.28

240. Malec, J., Harvey, R. F. & Cayner, J. J. Cannabis effect on spasticity in spinal cord injury. *Arch. Phys. Med. Rehabil.* **63**, 116–118 (1982).

241. Cardenas, D. D. & Jensen, M. P. Treatments for chronic pain in persons with spinal cord injury: a survey study. *J. Spinal Cord Med.* **29**, 109–117 (2006).

242. Warms, C. A., Turner, J. A., Marshall, H. M. & Cardenas, D. D. Treatments for chronic pain associated with spinal cord injuries: many are tried, few are helpful. *Clin. J. Pain* **18**, 154–163 (2011).

243. Heutink, M., Post, M. W. M., Wollaars, M. M. & van Asbeck, F. W. A. Chronic spinal cord injury pain: pharmacological and non-pharmacological treatments and treatment effectiveness. *Disabil. Rehabil.* **33**, 433–440 (2011). doi:10.3109/09638288.2010.498557

244. Teasell, R. W. *et al.* A systematic review of pharmacologic treatments of pain after spinal cord injury. *Arch. Phys. Med. Rehabil.* **91**, 816–831 (2010). doi:10.1016/j.apmr.2010.01.022

245. Arevalo-Martin, A. *et al.* Early endogenous activation of CB1 and CB2 receptors after spinal cord injury is a protective response involved in spontaneous recovery. *PLoS One* **7**, e49057 (2012). doi:10.1371/journal.pone.0049057

246. Kumar, A., Trescher, W. & Byler, D. Tourette syndrome and comorbid neuropsychiatric conditions. *Curr. Dev. Disord. Reports* **3**, 217–221 (2016). doi:10.1007/s40474-016-0099-1

247. Jakubovski, E., Müller-Vahl, K., Jakubovski, E. & Müller-Vahl, K. Speechlessness in Gilles de la Tourette syndrome: cannabis-based medicines improve severe vocal blocking tics in two patients. *Int. J. Mol. Sci.* **18**, 1739 (2017). doi:10.3390/ijms18081739

248. Abi-Jaoude, E., Chen, L., Cheung, P., Bhikram, T. & Sandor, P. Preliminary evidence on cannabis effectiveness and tolerability for adults with Tourette syndrome. *J. Neuropsychiatry Clin. Neurosci.* **29**, 391–400 (2017). doi:10.1176/appi.neuropsych.16110310

249. Kanaan, A. S., Jakubovski, E. & Müller-Vahl, K. Significant tic reduction in an otherwise treatment-resistant patient with Gilles de la Tourette syndrome following treatment with nabiximols. *Brain Sci.* **7**, 47 (2017). doi:10.3390/brainsci7050047

250. Skaper, S. D. & Di Marzo, V. Endocannabinoids in nervous system health and disease: the big picture in a nutshell. *Philos. Trans. R. Soc. London Ser. B, Biol. Sci.* **367**, 3193–3200 (2012). doi:10.1098/rstb.2012.0313

251. Mishima, K. *et al.* Cannabidiol prevents cerebral infarction via a serotonergic 5-hydroxytryptamine1A receptor–dependent mechanism. *Stroke* **36**, 1077–1082 (2005). doi:10.1161/01.STR.0000163083.59201.34

252. Mechoulam, R., Panikashvili, D. & Shohami, E. Cannabinoids and brain injury: therapeutic implications. *Trends Mol. Med.* **8**, 58–61 (2002).

253. Lopez-Rodriguez, A. B. *et al.* CB1 and CB2 cannabinoid receptor antagonists prevent minocycline-induced neuroprotection following traumatic brain injury in mice. *Cereb. Cortex* **25**, 35–45 (2015). doi:10.1093/cercor/bht202

254. Shohami, E., Cohen-Yeshurun, A., Magid, L., Algali, M. & Mechoulam, R. Endocannabinoids and traumatic brain injury. *Br. J. Pharmacol.* **163**, 1402–1410 (2011). doi:10.1111/j.1476-5381.2011.01343.x

255. Hazekamp, A. & Heerdink, E. R. The prevalence and incidence of medicinal cannabis on prescription in The Netherlands. *Eur. J. Clin. Pharmacol.* **69**, 1575–1580 (2013). doi:10.1007/s00228-013-1503-y

256. Zolotov, Y., Baruch, Y., Reuveni, H. & Magnezi, R. Adherence to medical cannabis among licensed patients in Israel. *Cannabis Cannabinoid Res.* **1**, 16–21 (2016). doi:10.1089/can.2015.0003

257. de Hoop, B., Heerdink, E. R. & Hazekamp, A. Medicinal cannabis on prescription in The Netherlands: statistics for 2003–2016. *Cannabis Cannabinoid Res.* **3**, 54–55 (2018). doi:10.1089/can.2017.0059

258. Government of Canada. *Cannabis Market Data.* (2018). Available at: https://www.canada.ca/en/health-canada/services/drugs-medication/cannabis/licensed-producers/market-data.html

259. Walsh, Z. *et al.* Cannabis for therapeutic purposes: patient characteristics, access, and reasons for use. *Int. J. Drug Policy* **24**, 511–516 (2013). doi:10.1016/j.drugpo.2013.08.010

260. Wilsey, B. *et al.* Low-dose vaporized cannabis significantly improves neuropathic pain. *J. Pain* **14**, 136–148 (2013).

261. Zuurman, L., Ippel, A. E., Moin, E. & van Gerven, J. M. A. Biomarkers for the effects of cannabis and THC in healthy volunteers. *Br. J. Clin. Pharmacol.* **67**, 5–21 (2009). doi:10.1016/j.jpain.2012.10.009

262. Romano, E. & Voas, R. B. Drug and alcohol involvement in four types of fatal crashes. *J. Stud. Alcohol Drugs* **72**, 567–576 (2011). doi:10.15288/jsad.2011.72.567